I DISAGREE

How These Two Words are the
Secret to Thinking Differently and
Taking Control of Your Health

DR. PATRICK FLYNN

Published by Best Seller Publishing®, Pasadena, CA

Best Seller Publishing® is a registered trademark

Printed in the United States of America.

ISBN 978-1-095315-23-1

This publication is designed to provide accurate and authoritative information with regard to the subject matter covered. It is sold with the understanding that the publisher is not engaged in rendering legal, accounting, or other professional advice. If legal advice or other expert assistance is required, the services of a competent professional should be sought. The opinions expressed by the authors in this book are not endorsed by Best Seller Publishing® and are the sole responsibility of the author rendering the opinion.

Most Best Seller Publishing® titles are available at special quantity discounts for bulk purchases for sales promotions, premiums, fundraising, and educational use. Special versions or book excerpts can also be created to fit specific needs.

For more information, please write:

Best Seller Publishing®

1346 Walnut Street, #205

Pasadena, CA 91106

or call 1(626) 765 9750

Toll Free: 1(844) 850-3500

Visit us online at: www.BestSellerPublishing.org

Table of Contents

Acknowledgments

I want to offer a very special appreciation to the core writing team that put his book together—Dawn, Renée, and my wife, Christy. Your commitment, long hours, and dedication brought this dream into reality! For that, I thank you.

The influence for this project came from far and wide. At The Wellness Way, we truly have an Us, We, Our Culture. Pieces of everyone's stories woven together—doctors and patients alike, all contributing to the movement, the momentum, and the impact that is changing lives. Thank you to each and every individual who has joined us in thinking differently. Together we are making a difference, and improving the health of people around the world!

Dedication

To my beautiful bride, Christy:

I choose you.

A Note From The Author

We've all had those moments. Maybe it hits you in the shower, or maybe it runs through your mind while you're driving. It definitely hits you when your opinionated cousin won't stop talking at the family reunion! It's the thought that something is wrong. Maybe you can't even put your finger on it, but you know something isn't right. You know you disagree with what's happening.

We all know a couple who is desperate for a baby. They've spent tens of thousands of dollars on treatments, but there is still no child. Maybe the couple is even you. The money invested is overwhelming, but the heartache even more so. Let me ask you a question though… why is this so common?

We all have the stories. Remember a time when you looked into a loved one's eyes, only to hear that the doctors said surgery is the only answer. Or another prescription was going to be written to see if it might help. Or even how they were told that despite the obvious symptoms, there was nothing wrong with them. Remember how you felt? In spite of everything, did a voice in your head whisper "no"?

Every day the news stations are flooded with reports of how people are sicker than ever. How can we have the best medical technologies and research, and people are STILL on an average of at least 4 prescriptions a day, NOT including the over-the-counter medications they take? How many prescriptions does a person need to be healthy?

Here's one more question for you: when is enough, enough? Would you agree that this is the best we have to offer ourselves, or would you disagree?

Let me answer first: I disagree. You disagree too, or you wouldn't be reading this book. Maybe you're not even sure what the answer is, but want to learn more. Awesome – let me be the first to welcome you to the family.

What you are going to find in this book is a different way of thinking. A way of thinking that is changing the lives of people across the country, giving them hope, and getting them results they never dreamed they could have. I hope you laugh, but you might cry, and you might even get upset – guess what? That's ok. Hang in there with me. This book is something you'll hear nowhere else, and sometimes it takes some time to work through something new. It will be valuable though – I promise!

Saying, "I Disagree," will be the most powerful thing you can learn to do. It's not destructive, in fact, when done based on facts and not emotions, it can be the most constructive thing a person can do! This book will show you why, and how. I'm excited and grateful to bring you the information our clinics across the country share with their patients every day. Disagree with a thought process that doesn't work! Disagree with a health care system that is clearly broken! Disagree with shattered hope, take a stand, and think differently!

Brenda's Story

Dr. Patrick has been instrumental in helping me understand the proper approach to healthcare instead of our current system. I met him after dealing with a health problem that had me seeing several doctors and specialists, visiting many emergency rooms, and on an overall path that was leading me down a spiral toward further disease and illness. I was honestly starting to wonder how much longer I could function at my current lifestyle pace. I felt like I was starting to lose my grip on my reality.

He is passionate about his calling. It was evident from the first time I met him. He took time to understand my story and concerns, ordered labs, and offered key nutritional changes that identified the underlying cause of my condition and allowed my body to take the steps needed for proper healing. He is an absolute visionary when it comes to the immune system, hormones, and understanding the biological root cause behind the symptoms. He helped me pull the pieces of the puzzle together and empowered me to take control to create a path that I didn't even know existed.

Dr. Patrick is also a genius at the biochemistry involved at the intersection between stress and illness. My life has been transformed by the knowledge of how stress impacts my hormones. This understanding has helped me slow the chatter of mind and pace of my life by giving me the ability to witness and understand the biological response to stressful situations. He helped me understand the chemicals involved in stress and the damage that can result to my hormones and body. I was able to see for the first time that my power lies in my response to any situation or perceived problem. I can control the stress reaction by simply becoming aware of it. I came to him with a health problem that he not only helped me restore but he also helped me find my power. Talk about transformation! I am beyond fortunate to have him in my life and am honored to be able to watch him change the lives of those around me.

CHAPTER 1

Everybody Has a Story

Everyone has a story. Every demographic, every walk of life. Regardless of who or what or when, what is common to all of us is that we each have a story. Each story is unique, and each story is important. They shape who we are, who we become, and collectively our stories impact what happens in our generation and for generations to come.

As you go through the journey of your life, *your story*, you encounter circumstances and situations that change you. It's part of the process, and an important part of determining how you think and look at the world. It can happen directly, or indirectly – sometimes you learn from things you go through yourself, and other times the experiences of others can have a tremendous effect.

Throughout this book, I'm going to share pieces of my story. Some parts may seem distant to you, while others may resonate so strongly that you see yourself in the scene. I have learned from things I've gone through myself, as well as things I've watched others experience. It has all led to thinking differently. Thinking in a way that has empowered myself and others to make lasting changes in their story. Changes that seemed impossible. Changes for the good.

This first story is a doozy of a story and one that shaped me more than I could ever imagine. I met a girl that I fell in love with and I fell hard! We knew mutual acquaintances who had tried to set us up on blind dates months before, but we both had bailed. I was busy with school is my excuse. But nineteen years ago, God orchestrated a chain of events that would change my life forever. I will *never* forget the day I met her. During the summer, I was a water-skier for a show ski team from my hometown of Crivitz. One day the pyramid fell on me and I gashed my cheek. I also had a mild concussion, so I went to get adjusted by a chiropractic buddy I used

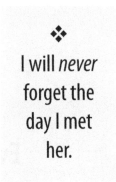

❖
I will *never* forget the day I met her.

to intern with. While I was there, a beautiful young lady with blond hair, short shorts, long legs and platform heels came in without an appointment. We were introduced and hit it off immediately! I learned later this was the SAME girl that I was set up on blind dates with; the ones we had both bailed on. (Crazy, right?)

Two days later we started dating. No joke! She told me, "I'm going to marry you someday," and I told her, "you're right!" There was something amazing and unique about this girl. We spent the first couple weeks of our relationship sharing our hearts and what we each wanted for our lives. She shared her dreams; I shared my vision and direction for my life. We discussed the family we wanted to have, where we wanted to live, our passions and goals. We also shared how we would raise our children and the ways we wanted to make a difference in the world. Remember, we were young. My career was just getting started. We had the whole world ahead of us.

Two weeks into our relationship, I went to her house excited to see the beautiful woman I had fallen in love with. When I got there, she was sobbing and in pain. This wouldn't be the last time I would find her like this. In the coming months, I would find her on the floor curled up in pain. It crushed me to see her like this. I wanted to know what I could do to help.

I would do anything for her. This wasn't just any girl–this was THE girl! So…why was she sobbing? I thought things were going so well. She had gotten her period that day, leaving her crying and in tremendous pain. I had no idea she had so much pain in her life. She was always so happy. There was more to this story than just female problems or hormone issues. In order to understand the big picture of what was really happening, let's step back a bit in "the girl's" life and health history.

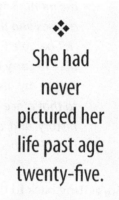

She had never pictured her life past age twenty-five.

Christy had struggled most of her life with various illnesses and conditions, and they got progressively worse as she entered college. Years later she told me that before we met, she had never pictured her life past age twenty-five. That's how sick she was.

CHRISTY'S THOUGHTS:

What was I thinking that day when Patrick found me sobbing and in pain?

Why would a guy like him–someone so confident, bold and driven to achieve his future goals and dreams–want to be with a girl like me? You see, I was sick and had had many health challenges throughout my life up to that point. We had already talked about what we dreamed our futures would look like. I honestly didn't know what my future would look like, because doctors had given me a grim outlook. I had excruciating GI issues including ulcerative colitis that was on the road to becoming Crohn's. The medical doctor's best advice at the time was, "drink Maalox before and after every meal." Seriously? I did that, and I was so much worse! All they could offer me were more drugs and later on surgery would be inevitable. To me that was crazy!

> Around that same time period (while I was in college), my reproductive issues also began to take over my life. From migraines to incredible cramping, I felt like every organ of my body was slowly shutting down. The doctors and specialists monitored my symptoms and then suggested drugs. I refused the drugs, so they insisted on monitoring me monthly with ultrasounds. They confirmed that I had cysts on my ovaries and that I had endometriosis. They told me I would probably not be able to bear children, or if I were to conceive, I would not be able to carry the pregnancy to term. Then they graciously offered to scrape my uterus. I politely said, 'no thank you,' and never returned to that office again. My mom had shared other details of my health history, and, as a result, I was at peace with the fact that I might not be able to bear my own children. I could definitely adopt some day.

So, getting back to this pivotal, emotional moment in our lives, Christy began to share with me for the first time the health struggles that she had endured. I didn't know any of this until I found her in pain. I was shocked she was struggling like this. She even went so far as to say, "maybe we shouldn't be together." Now, I had a decision to make. While we had been sharing our hearts in that fantastic first two weeks of our relationship, I had shared with her I wanted a big family. So, I had a choice to make right then and there. Do I stay with her or do I leave her? I'm not kidding when I told you I had completely fallen head-over-heels for that beautiful woman. Do I chalk this up as a set back? Or, do I choose to use it as a set up for one of the greatest gifts God has ever given me?

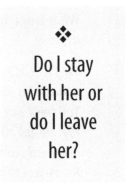

❖

Do I stay with her or do I leave her?

Because I loved Christy and we had a future in front of us we both clearly wanted, the choice was obvious. The choice was her; it was us. It was easy to choose us because I had fallen madly in love. She asked,

"But what about your dream of having children? The doctors say I might never be able to give you a child."

When I looked at that beautiful woman that I loved, I realized that there were two words that would define our future. I disagree. I disagree with every doctor she saw. *I disagree* with the general practitioners. I disagree with the gynecologists. I disagree with the specialists. I even disagree with the chiropractor who was giving her regular adjustments and great supplements. The beautiful woman I fell in love with was meant to have children just like every other woman. There was something they were all missing. I didn't know what it was, but I was determined to find out.

I engulfed myself into the study of female hormones. I devoured everything I could find, every research article, every study, everything. I spoke with other doctors I respected, people who had been my instructors while I was in school and others who had a mindset to look at things differently. I wanted to see multiple perspectives and put the pieces together. I studied female hormones like a fanatic. The best answers I found were disheartening. All I could think was: *Man, this can't be all there is!* I knew this didn't line up with what I had been taught in school. I couldn't settle for what I was finding. I knew there was more to it. I had to keep digging and look at it from a different approach. I had to think differently.

Just because we have what appears to be a fairytale life doesn't mean it was easy. We had obstacles. Every decision you make will have obstacles. The question is, will you overcome the obstacles to get to the end you want?

CHRISTY'S THOUGHTS:

Some people say they wish they knew exactly what obstacles they would face in life so they could prepare. In my case, if I had known how hard my journey was going to be, I don't think I would've had enough courage to walk it. By the grace of God, I was introduced to a man I fell in love with and he turned my world upside down. For so long I felt alone in my health journey. Appointment after appointment I kept hearing the same two things: "We aren't sure why" and "here are some drugs and surgery to help your pain." I was discouraged to say the least-even a bit depressed at times. The medical method was getting me nowhere, and I kept feeling worse. I couldn't eat typical healthy foods like salad, certain fruits and vegetables, and I had been allergic to dairy since the second grade. I had been seen and referred to so many doctors, but no one could give any answers on how to become healthy. I was exhausted and ready to try something different. So, imagine me on the floor crying, being vulnerable with Patrick for the first time. I was so afraid of what was going to come next. But then he said something that no one ever said to me before. "Don't worry about any of this. You're going to be okay." I chose at that very moment to trust him-a guy I just met-with my health and future. How crazy is THAT?!? I knew that this road was not going to be easy to travel, but the medical model had nothing to offer me that made sense. I chose to trust the process of the journey we were going to be walking together.

We chose to stay with it no matter what, including all the criticisms that come when living under a microscope.

I may have been a new doctor, but I was convinced a woman's body was meant to have babies. You see, I believe all bodies are created for homeostasis. Homeostasis is health and function. That was more than any other doctor had offered her. I chose to look at things differently and not settle for the answers she had been given. This unfamiliar approach was foreign to both of our families, and as a result, caused stress and struggles within our relationships. We chose to stay with it no matter what, including all the criticisms that come when living under a microscope. What's the result? What was the impact of our decision to pursue Christy's health? We have four amazing daughters. Yes, I have FOUR daughters. You can please all pray for me now! I joke, but they are amazing and bring so much joy to our lives. Sometimes I wonder what my life would have been like if I hadn't chosen Christy. If we hadn't disagreed with what the traditional medical thinking offered. I know it wouldn't be as amazing as life with Christy and these four girls.

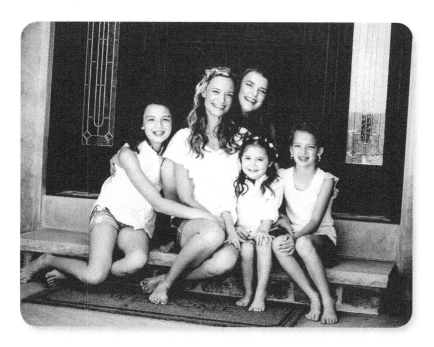

There's another huge impact from that original choice to pursue a different understanding of health. One I hadn't known at the time when Christy and I chose to build a future together; a result that has impacted men, women, and children all over the world. It was a change of thought process. I had to look at things from a different approach and not just settle for the "one size fits all" method the traditional medical world uses. Now others are learning to ask questions and think differently. That is a big deal for a culture that historically never questioned anyone in a white coat; they are the experts. There is a lot of power in those two words, I disagree. More people are saying it because of the decisions my wife and I made almost twenty years ago. If you think about it, that is a big impact. Much bigger than we could have imagined at that time.

Actually, a huge national company impacting thousands of people around the world every year would not exist if I hadn't chosen my wife. The Wellness Way wouldn't be where it is today if I hadn't chosen Christy and her unique health. This pivotal change of thought process impacted my wife and created the opportunity for us to have a family with those four amazing daughters. Now I'm using our experience to help families all over the world. I'm here to empower you in your choices; they have an impact. My impact all started with a change in thought process. But I'm getting ahead of myself. Let me tell you about what I learned, and you can decide for yourself.

Is Common Normal?

I have some simple questions for you. Don't worry, I'll help you along with the answers. Would you agree in the past 30 years we have more hospitals? That's obvious. More doctors? There's a specialist for everything! Spend more money on health care? We spend more on health care than ever before and our country spends more than any other country! Do we have more medications? Yes! The average American is on four to seven medications. We also have more medical interventions than ever before. With so much more medicine you would think we would be the healthiest people on the planet. But do you know what many of them consider the best solution for addressing female hormone concerns? Horse urine. I had to keep studying, so I kept reading and researching.

The stuff I found was mind blowing. Let me ask you a question. If you have a daughter, when she gets to her teenage years, she's going to go through a change in life, correct? It's called puberty and it's natural. It happens to every young woman. Yet, there are times when the evidence of puberty (the menstrual cycle) is inconvenient, so the medical approach looks for "solutions" to these natural phases of life. Here was an interesting article I found. Horse hormone given to young women to stop them from having a menstrual cycle. I found this article in a very popular "health" magazine. The article starts: "Sick of your period? Get rid of it!" I read the article and thought, *maybe this is the thing, maybe they have it right. Perhaps women don't need a cycle.* At the University of Florida Health Sciences Medical School, with the assistance of medication, doctors have now agreed that cycles are optional. But only with the help of a medication. I started to research this idea further and I found that doctors believe there is no medical reason to menstruate. Ever. I had to read what the medication does to make this possible, because this obviously wasn't a natural process. The prescribed medication causes the uterine lining to harden so you won't have a period anymore. However, underneath everything still works.

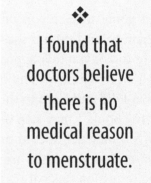

I found that doctors believe there is no medical reason to menstruate.

What do you think this causes the uterus to do? Like a balloon, it gets bigger and bigger until it actually explodes. The doctors agreed this is not dangerous, however, it may be inconvenient. I'm sure they have their reasoning for that thought, but ladies, if your uterus explodes, is that a little bit more than inconvenient?

I spent time reading thousands of articles by the best doctors in their field and this was the best I could find. This was the only thing they had for my wife. How frustrating this must be for you ladies. After all my reading and research, after seeing hundreds of women a year for eighteen years, I can speak with great confidence on one thing. You want to know what it is? I thank God every day that I don't have a vagina. Every day. Guys, we are pretty lucky and have it pretty easy. We really do. I also started to realize women didn't understand their own bodies. My wife at that time was twenty-three years old and had no clue. Many women today have no clue what is going on with their bodies. They don't understand men and their hormones, and men don't understand their own hormones nor those of their partners. The medical treatment women are getting is a strong indicator that the traditional thinking is failing all of us. I think it's time for all of us to look beyond what we may have been told. It's time for more people to disagree.

I'm going to take you on a path, so you can see for yourself how I began to understand these hormones and functions and how we are able to convey this approach in offices all over the country. To take you on this journey and bring understanding, I need to get you to do what I did and learn to think differently. It will set the stage for the rest of the book. I may step on some toes through this process, and some of you may get uncomfortable. That's not my goal, but I understand sometimes new paths are uncomfortable. Please trust me when I say the results on this path are worth it!

Think about some of the statistics we see daily. Now versus any time in history, do we have more or less heart disease? More or less cancer? More or less fertility problems? If we keep on that same thinking, most of you will have the same situations as everybody else. Just because something is common does not mean it's normal. I want to help you so that you will start thinking

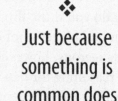

Just because something is common does not mean it's normal.

differently. To get you to think differently, I have to come up with an altered approach. That is what I and a growing group of doctors are calling The Wellness Way Approach. With the increase in medical advancement should we really have more cancer, more infertility, more autoimmune issues, more heart disease and more unhealthy people? Many people think because it is common that it's normal. By the end of this book I want you to disagree.

A Note from Christy:

On being the first patient of The Hormone Whisperer:

I'm just a small-town country girl who fell in love with an amazing small-town guy. He had a vision in his heart to help people regain their health. I'm honored to have been his first patient in this way and to see where it has led. It's overwhelming to think I had some small part in that. I remember the day Patrick came to my place and I was on the floor in a fetal position. There were a lot of emotions.

I remember him just brushing it off when I told him I was probably not going to be able to have children. He said, "I disagree, don't worry." I figured we would cross that bridge when we got there. He was so sure, and I trusted in that.

Patrick was the only person willing to connect the dots for me. He was the only person who bothered to look for a solution. He gave me hope. I had learned enough to know I wanted to do things naturally. I was already under chiropractic care, but what I didn't know was the power of chiropractic care. Many people only think of chiropractic care as pain management for physical trauma. There is a whole philosophy of chiropractic relating to the 3T's (thoughts, toxins and trauma) unknown to so many people. Once I understood where true health came from and how to regain homeostasis, there was no turning back. I met Patrick and I never stepped foot into another OB/GYN's office. That was it. I was all-in. I never looked back. He practiced adjusting on me. He took me to all his chiropractor friends who had graduated before him, I was adjusted by all of them including doctors with whom he had interned. Patrick was determined to figure out why my body was so sick and to return it to normal. We both disagreed and now he had to teach me how to think differently.

We did some dramatic things such as eliminating sugar completely from our lives! I remember the day like it was yesterday. I cried. I was emotionally addicted. My mother and grandmother had taught me to bake. It was how we showed love and care for our family. I had to make a decision; to be healthy or remain sick. Now, years later, I love to create new recipes using healthier ingredients comparable to those treats from long ago in the kitchens of my childhood. It's not easy. You have to make a choice. Treat everything you put into your mouth as either bringing life or bringing death.

Patrick proposed to me outside of a new hospital. I imagine this may not sound like the traditional engagement story, but it is a huge part of our story. We were walking the quiet path on the hospital grounds with the soft lights and large snowflakes falling around us. I didn't truly understand at that point. Can anyone really understand what is to come? It was romantic in our way. I understood his heart, his dreams and vision. I knew as long as we would walk through it together, it would be worth it. He was proposing to the woman he loved in front of the paradigm and dogma he battled. He told me if I agreed to be with him for the rest of our lives, it would include a journey-an uphill battle. Patrick wanted me to know I was saying yes to not only him, but this life. I knew no matter how hard it would get or what the adversities we faced, it would all be worth it.

When he proposed to me, did I have any inkling that our life would look anything like it does? No! Oh, my goodness, no! When I was a kid and dreamed of my life, I never dream past age 25. I would never dream about marriage or life past that point. Ironic, we got married when I was 25 and my life completely changed. I couldn't have pictured it if I had tried.

In the beginning this new life was a struggle. I lived on an island for many years, going against the grain. No one was doing what we were doing. As the years went by we built a community of people, educating and inspiring them to become healthier and to create healthy families. We created the community we needed right in Green Bay, Wisconsin. The dynamics of our city changed. We had patients go to the grocery store requesting healthier ingredients eliminating the need to have to drive to Milwaukee on a regular basis just to stock our pantries. This community of people who used to be sick and unhealthy became a transforming group of like-minded individuals. They were taking a stand for what was needed for their own health and their families.

When we were ready to start our family with children and stopped trying to "not get pregnant," I got pregnant right away. I was so excited. We told people right away. We didn't live in fear. We didn't seek the hospital route. Instead, we chose to have our sweet and precious babies at home with a midwife.

Don't allow someone to tell you it's not possible. Don't allow someone to try to scare you or make you believe lies. God created us to be mothers. We need to support and encourage each other. We need to reinforce this within a broken healthcare paradigm. There is a different way—The Wellness Way. This is the pathway to create a healthy family. We need to ask a different question to find the answers we need. What isn't functioning correctly? Why isn't it functioning correctly? Be willing to approach hurdles in a different way than you have before. You may be amazed at the people who come across your path who have the answers to the prayers you've prayed.

I'm excited for the many people who can be helped by this approach. This is about getting results. The principles and testing allow us to give people hope, answers, and the ability to see things differently. Patrick always talks about the importance of being able to step back and approach your challenges with a different mindset. The Wellness Way approach is an idea – an idea that says we are not genetically programmed for disease or illness, but for health. It's based on the philosophy that you can only truly be healthy if you address all 3T's. We test because everyone is unique and should be treated that way. How are these 3T's affecting you specifically? They focus on who you are and what you need; not a standard procedure.

This book and seminar help people look at all healthcare options. If we could do that for one person, it has all been worth it. The best part is in knowing so many people can be helped. After Patrick started helping me, women began coming from all over. They included a friend my age who was prescribed pre-menopausal drugs, to others who were given no choice but to take some form of artificial hormone. Word travels fast. Now women are calling from all over the world. I've been able to watch as Patrick has been able to offer different answers to so many women. He's given hope to those who want to bear children, building their own legacy and future family, while impacting their children's children. Raising those healthy kids is another whole adventure! We are creating a healthier society, one baby and momma at a time.

Looking forward, I'm excited to create a different legacy of thought. I don't fear my girls not having babies. I'm excited. I talk to our girls about having children and a large family if they choose. It is joyous to discuss bringing life into the world and doing what God has called us to do as women. He's given us gifts to do what men cannot. The gift to be mothers. I want my girls to embrace it. To know that being a mother is a blessing. A gift. It's something to be celebrated and not treated as if it were a disease to be fixed or medicated.

I'm very proud of the man Patrick has become and I'm excited to see how God continues to use him. I'm blessed to be on this journey with him and I can't imagine life without him. He's affected so many people and I'm inspired by that man's brain, but most of all his heart. Of course, he's good looking, but ultimately, talking with him; the way his brain works is so intriguing. I could listen to him teach all day. I wanted to marry an intelligent and intriguing man. I love learning from him and how we look at the future-learning, growing and continuing on this journey together. My husband is the most generous, honest, and caring man. He never stops researching. He seeks out the best quality labs and products to ensure the greatest results in all the clinics across the country. The only variable is what you will choose.

ON THE TO DO LISTS:

As he was coming up with the To Do Lists, Patrick started telling me about the things I was doing to help our marriage. I wasn't even aware that I was following a To Do List! Every once in a while, I'll gauge myself to make sure I'm keeping up with my end of the To Do Lists. Even though I helped to create them, I know I need to stay mindful to continue with them for our marriage. They can change a marriage. I know what marriage is like before the To Do Lists and the results once they are implemented. Every marriage has struggles but having useful tools helps point the way to a better marriage. Use the tools and the To Do Lists. Both the husband and the wife need to come to a point where they are humble enough to recognize the needs of the other person need to come first and be met. We need to recognize we don't have to be the same. Patrick and I are two totally different people. When you respect and recognize each other's differences, celebrate and embrace them, an amazing marriage can be built. When women complain and nag, I just want to pull them aside and tell them they don't understand their husband. Likewise, a husband shouldn't be stressing his wife. He may not understand that he is causing her to stress and in doing so depleting her hormones. It's a two-way street. If a husband and a wife can humble themselves and honestly look at what they need to change in their own behaviors and actions, it's a recipe for a better relationship.

Ladies, I encourage you, your partner may not want to read the book (his hormones may not let him sit still that long). He will love the seminar. He will enjoy the entertaining approach. You'll leave with real tools to put to work right away. Get you and your husband to a seminar. Almost every woman who comes to the seminar without her husband tells us, "I wish I would have brought my husband!" If you are looking for answers or highly entertaining information, you'll find it at The Hormone Connection seminar. It's a fresh perspective and look at a topic that affects every man, woman and family. Check in with your nearest Wellness Way clinic for The Hormone Connection seminar schedule. It will change your life.

When a partner can gain insight into their marriage and what could be going on physiologically, hopelessness is born into new hope. This isn't just a story. This is the dedication and passion of our life. This is our real-life story. I believe it gives hope.

This man is the love of my life. He's the incredible father of our four beautiful girls. From daily dance parties when daddy gets home each night, to watching an occasional romantic "chick flick" with me snuggled on the couch – he always puts us first no matter how busy he gets.

CLOSING THOUGHTS:

I love our story. I love that Patrick is so passionate about hormones and the irony that we have four girls! We have a new legacy of mommas. I'm thankful and grateful for what God has given me: my husband, my children and to be a part of this story that has come to change so many people's lives. It's overwhelming.

Daily, I'm on my knees praying for my husband and The Wellness Way. We are on a quest to continue the relentless pursuit of doing the right thing and getting the information out to the people. We will continue regardless of what comes our way; regardless of the hate mail and regardless of obstacles. One of the biggest lessons I've learned and wish to pass on to you, dear reader: Don't let your future be dictated by someone else's fear.

Chapter 2

Firemen and Carpenters

My wife went to many practitioners over the years before I met her. She saw obstetricians, gastrointestinal specialists, neurologists, chiropractors, a naturopath and so many others in her search for help. They each had their own answers for her. The medical doctors prescribed drugs and suggested scraping out her uterus. She knew that wasn't her answer. Christy looked at the side effects and she knew she wanted a family one day. The natural doctors had her on a ton of supplements that cost her a lot of money. She was taking all of those supplements when I met her! She was trying to do everything right, but she still felt worse. She couldn't eat a salad because her digestion was so messed up, and I found her crying in the fetal position on the first day of her period. How do you think she would have felt five years later? Or ten years later? She would have been very sick, because up until now we have only had one mindset. I'm going to let you in on what is different about our mindset.

How many of you have sat in a doctor's office and been told that there is nothing they can do for you. Or what they can do for you is a drug with a bunch of side effects. You might have also been told that there is nothing wrong with you. Even though you have a laundry list of symptoms, they might not be able to find a diagnosis—so there is nothing they can do for you. That is one of the worst feelings a person can have. To feel trapped by illness with the only answers from the "experts" leaving you further trapped.

Anyone who knows me, knows that I love to create analogies and use them frequently. Why? We've all sat with doctors, looked at them, they've looked at us, and we made sure that we were listening. We even told them we understood what they were saying! Then when we left the appointment and thought, "what in the world did they just say?" The doctor sounded very smart but didn't connect with you. You had no clue what you were doing, and you were taking him or her on faith. I find analogies are much easier to remember than "doctor speak"!

That is one of the worst feelings a person can have. To feel trapped by illness with the only answers from the "experts" leaving you further trapped.

Let me give you an example. Before I sit down with a woman, I go through the list of medications she is taking. If a woman is taking something like Premarin, I ask her if she has an affinity for carrots. Why do I ask her that? Most people don't know that Premarin comes from **preg**nant **mar**e ur**ine**. It's a funny question, but I'm trying to get her to think differently. When they look at me confused, I say "Well, you are putting horse urine into your body and they like carrots and sugar cane, so I was just wondering." Women are stunned when they learn what has really been prescribed to them. They should know though. Would you agree that if a woman has been given a horse hormone and doesn't know it, she should be upset? Absolutely. I don't have a problem with someone taking something as long as they know what they are taking, what it is doing, why they are taking it, for how long they will be taking it, and all the effects that go along with that plan.

Let me share the analogy that has set the foundation for everything since I started. It sets the basis for every patient that we work with. I believe if you understand this simple analogy, you will understand which doctor to use. Some of you are reading this book because you are frustrated with your doctor. Especially now that you have started to change your thinking. This is something I want to make sure you read closely. I'm not saying you shouldn't go back, I'm saying you should know *why* and *when* to go back. By the time we are done here, I want you to be able to have a clearer understanding of health, and be confident in your choices. I want you to know when to say, "I disagree," and when to let them save your life.

Firemen and Carpenters

Let's say you've been out for a nice dinner with your family and you get home to find your house on fire. Who is the best professional to handle this situation? A fireman. Why wouldn't you call your dentist? Doesn't he have a hose? That question probably made you grin. You're thinking, *Doc, that's a silly question!* Well, it's a silly question because you know that if he showed up with his tools, and his hose, he could get himself killed. The fireman is the best trained professional to handle the situation.

So, let's walk through the scenario. The fire truck pulls up and the firemen basically have two tools to work with; hoses and axes. With the ax, the firefighter runs up to your house where he crashes your door in and then smashes the windows. The guy with the hose then runs in and starts spraying the inside of your house. Simple question, when the water he sprays hits the pictures of your kids, what does it do to them? The wall? What does it do to the carpet? The fire department has been there about fifteen minutes and what have they done to your house so far? You are standing there, grateful for all the different ways they have destroyed your home. All you'll have left is a burned-out shell of your home, and you are still grateful. Even though they caused massive

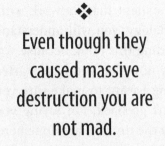

Even though they caused massive destruction you are not mad.

destruction you are not mad. Why? This is their job. But, can you live in that house? Is it toxic? Could it kill you? Let's remember, the fire department has done a good job and has done everything they were supposed to do with the knowledge and tools they have to work with. That doesn't mean your house is fit to live in.

A time will come when you've got to get back into your house. Who is the best professional to call now? The carpenter. Imagine the carpenter shows up while the fire department is still there. The carpenter sees a mess! He has to rip out walls and carpet and bring in the materials he needs to rebuild the house. Which person is right? Both; based on the specific need of the house at the specific time. If the carpenter shows up to the house while it's on fire, he looks like what? Now you might laugh at this question, because it's so obvious, but it illustrates my point! If he shows up with his tools of a hammer, nails, and lumber he looks really funny. Vice versa, if the fire department shows up and tries to rebuild the house with an ax and a hose, you would laugh again. Would you agree? Based on the need, you have to know which professional to call.

If you understand that example, you understand how healthcare should be run today. If you are having a stroke or heart attack, with the education you know that I have, should I run into your kitchen and grab a knife and see if I can help you? No! We need to call someone who is the best professional to save your life. Who are we going to call? We're going to call 9-1-1. For the purposes of the analogy, let's call traditional medicine the fire department. They're going to take you to the hospital and use their axes and hoses on you. Here's where some confusion comes in. When they put the hose into your arm and start pumping the medicine into your body, is it good for your body? Some say yes, and some say no. Let's go back to the example. When the fire department sprays water on the walls, is it good for the walls? You have to answer the question that was asked. I didn't ask if it saved your life. I didn't ask if it put out the fire. I asked if it was good for your body. If you look at the back of the medication bottle and the inserts, there are numerous warnings and negative side effects, and they are definitely not good for your body. The manufacturer presents this information. I'm not saying the medication is not needed, I'm just asking if it's good for you.

Now, let's say the medication didn't work. They only have one other tool; the ax. Could you possibly die from that surgery? Okay, can we come to an agreement? Could we agree that if you are having a heart attack, you may need drugs or surgery to stay alive? Even if they aren't necessarily good for your body, they are what is needed at the time to save the body from dying.

Let's go back to my wife. Did they give her medications when she presented her symptoms? If they are the fire department, they start with medication because it's how they can help her. The challenges my wife was dealing with would eventually develop into cancer. Then it would be time for the ax. They would tell her to have her uterus removed via hysterectomy. She went to some top specialists; but their way of thinking was the fire department. Do you follow me?

Let's look at the difference. Can you guess the number one reason why people have gone to the doctors in recent years? High blood pressure. Everybody knows someone with high blood pressure. Can someone die from high blood pressure? Yes! Do I have any problem with the fire department's approach using ACE inhibitors, channel blockers or

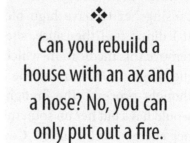

❖

Can you rebuild a house with an ax and a hose? No, you can only put out a fire.

Lasix? No, they save people's lives. But after the life has been saved, after all the warm thank-you's to the doctors and nurses, do they ever sit down with you and discuss why you've had the heart attack or stroke? Do they help you get your body back to healthy? They may suggest a bland diet and an occasional walk, but are they helping you to rebuild for a long and vibrant life? Can you rebuild a house with an ax and a hose? No, you can only put out a fire. Can you get your body back to normal with drugs or surgery? No, you can't. Today, we have fire department doctors. We need fire department doctors! But we also need carpenters. The Wellness Way Approach is the carpenter approach. I want to know what triggered your fire. We help our patients to repair the weak spots where fires can start, rebuild where fires have been, and best of all prevent any possible fires so that you can live that long and vibrant life!

When Christy presented me with these problems, I figured out what triggered her fires and how to rebuild her house. That's how we have four daughters today.

Let's take a look from another example in my office. What's the number one medication given for high blood pressure today? Many people take the medication Atenolol. Atenolol can save a life. I'm not saying it can't. But let's not forget a negative side effect is extreme fatigue. I had a woman come in with female hormone problems as well as extreme fatigue and thought I could help her. I looked at her medication list and told her I couldn't help her unless I found what was causing her to have high blood pressure.

If I didn't find the cause, she could never remove this medication-which was causing the fatigue! Do you see the difference in thought process? The firefighter approach would have put her on something to change her energy level, correct? Could that have worked? Yes, but now you've added another

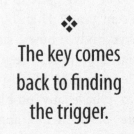

The key comes back to finding the trigger.

medication. If you watch TV or read ads in magazines, you will see medications competing over who can put out the fire faster. But they missed the point. I just ask a different question which is what caused the fire in the first place? The key comes back to finding the trigger.

I met my wife when I was almost done with chiropractic school but some of this story started even before that. You are probably assuming based on my success that I come from a wealthy family and was loved by all my teachers. That's not the case. Shortly after I married Christy, we ran into one of my old teachers at the grocery store. She didn't tell my beautiful bride that I was her favorite student. As I stood with my new bride by the frozen meats, my former teacher looked her dead in the eye and said, "I never thought he would become a doctor. I thought he'd end up in prison." My new wife looked at me with eyes that said, "What did I get myself into?"

I came from a hardworking family that worked to make the best for their children with what they had. My mom worked in a bank and had a second job as a waitress. My dad was a truck driver. I know that I was a hard child to raise and give them credit for doing all they could do. I was hypersensitive, my skin was always crawling, and I could never sit still. When the teacher said to work on a writing project, I was drawing a picture of myself hunting on the back. It was a very elaborate drawing, but I got a zero on that homework. I loved hunting, and I couldn't focus on the project my teacher wanted me to do. As the years went on it got worse. My mind was going a mile a minute. I could not sit still. Today they would have diagnosed me with ADHD and had me on a bunch of different drugs.

I see that today in my practice; they want to put children on drugs. I learned to think differently early on and now I can help kids who are going through what I went through. I know now that the body doesn't always need drugs, especially if we remove the trigger that is causing the problem. I now know I have an egg allergy that was triggering my system. If someone had looked at what was happening to my body and understood the approach I use now with my patients, it would have been a lot easier on my family. It would have been a lot easier on me. But I wouldn't be who I am today, which is someone who thinks differently.

A lot of people think because we think differently than the traditional medical approach that we are the natural approach. They get so excited when they see me. "Hey Doc, I totally get it. I don't take any medications and want to do things all natural." I reply, "Hold the phone. You're taking twenty supplements! What happens if you don't take those supplements?" They say, "Well, I can't poop." If you need to take a bunch of supplements to poop or feel normal, then you're still sick. You're still sick because the thinking of the popular natural movement and traditional medicine are the same. We have to change that thinking.

The natural movement will apply the same medical thinking to your symptoms but with natural remedies. The system of medicine leans toward acute care or treating the immediate problem or symptom. We call them firemen because they put out your immediate fire without addressing the rebuilding of the body. The natural approach has taken on that same thinking. Instead of giving you an ACE inhibitor for your high blood pressure, they treat your symptoms with fish oils, B12 shots, CoQ10, magnesium, potassium and other natural remedies. They are treating the symptoms instead of finding out why the body is displaying the symptom. One patient can have high blood pressure for a totally different reason than another.

The body doesn't make mistakes. If there is a symptom, there is a reason why the body is trying to adapt. It's not the symptom that you need to fix. You need to test and find out how to get your body to function. We aren't all the same. If you think of your neighbors, family members, or your spouse,

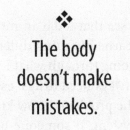

❖

The body doesn't make mistakes.

everybody is different. Why would applying the same medication, or natural treatment to everybody work for everyone? It wouldn't. That's why it's important to test to find out what is happening with the body. It doesn't make any sense to assume everybody needs the same thing and that just because it works for one person that it will work for everyone with those symptoms.

Who is the king of the natural movement? Dr. Oz! He is famous for this. Dr. Oz could put a one-armed man on his show and give him turmeric so that his arm grows back. When his arm grows back what happens with three million one-armed men the next day? They go out and buy turmeric. Boy, are they disappointed when their arms don't grow back. This is called the Dr. Oz Effect. I didn't make it up. Google it.

The Dr. Oz Effect is what happens when a product or treatment is featured on his show and tons of people rush out to try that product. Even though all these people are different and have diverse reasons for their symptoms. The Neti Pot was featured on the Dr. Oz Show and sales went up 12,000%! People searching for info on the Neti Pot went up 42,000%. Nobody ever searched raspberry ketones and green tea extract, but after mentions on the Dr. Oz show they are trending. The "King of Natural Remedies" always has something new to offer, and people rush to try it.

"But there are no side effects!" That's what I heard from a very upset natural practitioner after one of my talks. "At least with the natural movement you don't get the side effects of the medical system." She stumped me there for a bit, she was right. After a lot of thinking, I thought of one side effect—a smaller pocket book. You'll spend all that money on supplements but what will you get for it?

Which will fail first the medicine or natural remedy? The thing about treating symptoms with natural remedies is the natural remedy will fail first. A medical drug can force your body to do something. If you give a guy Viagra, his body will respond whether he wants it to or not. That doesn't happen with natural methods. You guys have heard this about natural remedies or had it happen to you. You took something, it helped for a little while, but then it stopped working. It didn't continue to work like it did in the beginning. It gave you false hope and then you're back on the medication you were on in the first place.

CHRISTY'S THOUGHTS

Before I met Patrick, I had tried just about everything. When I started to take some homeopathic tinctures and herbs, I felt a little better, but months and even years later I was still struggling with the same things; and if I didn't take my supplements–man, was I in excruciating pain! I'm sure there are many women who can relate to what I am saying. Anyone can push a certain product on you to try. At the end of the day, you need to ask how is this really making me healthier? It didn't make a difference what I took because I was asking the wrong questions. Instead of asking what can I take to make me healthy, I should have been asking what is not functioning? Where is my body deficient? How toxic am I?

That's why the natural movement and the Dr. Oz Effect are failing people. They take the same approach as the medical system, but it doesn't heal the body. It may (or may not) mask the symptoms for a while, but it doesn't get to addressing the body as a whole. That's why The Wellness Way Approach is different. We aren't the medical approach and we aren't the natural approach. We think differently.

I tested my wife from a different mindset. *I looked at what triggered her fire and asked how do I rebuild her body?* I didn't just balance my wife's hormones to get her pregnant four times, I got her body healthy. It's perfectly normal for a healthy woman to have a baby. That's a positive side effect! We don't test for fires, we test for what could trigger a fire and how to rebuild the house in such a way as to prevent that fire from

I didn't just balance my wife's hormones to get her pregnant four times, I got her body healthy.

ever occurring again. I know you didn't pick up this book to read about hormone issues. You really didn't. You were looking for something else, something that seems elusive. It's not. Stay with me. Let's talk about health and how we got here.

CHAPTER 3

What is Health?

When I look out at a crowd of people, I know they are looking for health. No matter what their job is or how big their house is, they all want health. At my seminars, I ask people to raise their hand if they want to be healthy. They don't just want health for themselves though. I ask if they want healthy kids, healthy parents and healthy in-laws. They all raise their hands that they want health for everyone they are close to.

The funny thing is very few people can tell me what "healthy" is. I hear a variety of answers and even a few responses of "I don't know." It makes sense. We've been taught about fires our whole lives. Fires like cancer, diabetes, heart disease, and all the others you see in drug commercials. Everybody wants to be healthy, but we know very little about it. How can you have something, or even want something, if you don't know what it is? That's why so many people are sick today.

Here's another question I ask people about health: What are three things that make you healthy?

I already know what they will say. We've been conditioned to think specific things make us healthy. Every audience answers the same way:

Food,

exercise,

and sleep.

These are the answers I hear every time. Just about everyone agrees these three things make you healthy. Unfortunately, it's yet another reason why people are so sick. These three things have very little to do with *making* you healthy. You know people who never eat well, never exercise, smoke every day and live to be 100 years old. George Burns lived to be 100 and we all know that he was very open with his cigars and martinis. Then you have people who simply come in contact with second-hand smoke and get cancer. Ladies, you know you hate those women who eat four donuts in the morning, never exercise and are thin. Why are they healthy even though they are eating unhealthy things and not exercising? But are they *really* healthy, or just thin?

You may be confused now and thinking food, exercise and sleep aren't important for you. I didn't say that. I asked you if that is where health *comes from*. They are very important to your health, but they aren't where health comes from. Just like when we talked about the house on fire, is putting the water on the walls good for the walls? We need to start thinking differently. If I hadn't learned to think differently, my beautiful bride would never have had four beautiful babies.

> ❖
> **Drugs and surgery have done a good job of keeping us alive.**

Let me give you an example from my office. I had a nurse practitioner from a local hospital visit me. She thought she had some hormone problems. We went through our normal exam. I took some x-rays and I saw a tumor. You know what I told her to do? I told her to go back to the hospital and check to make sure she wasn't going to die. Why? Can I rebuild the house if you are dead? No. They took a biopsy and decided since it wasn't going to grow so they'd just monitor it each year. That was the decision between her and her fire department-type doctor.

Let's say it was cancer and could have killed her. If they pulled it out, did they extend her life? Possibly. Did they make her healthy? No. Within two to five years she would very likely find herself with a new tumor. When you tell people from the "natural" side of healthcare the reason we live so long today is medicine, they tend to freak out. Drugs and surgery have done a good job of keeping us alive. They are doing their job. But we are still sick as dogs because they don't make us healthy.

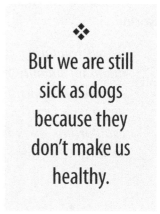

❖

But we are still sick as dogs because they don't make us healthy.

I don't like that definition of health where we are just being kept alive and treating symptoms, so I created one that I think is more accurate. Here's the definition of health we use at The Wellness Way:

A condition of wholeness in which all the organs are functioning 100% of the time.

Let's go back to the three healthy choices of food, exercise and sleep. Disregarding those conditions, if I cut my finger and my body is functioning well, it will heal. If my body is not functioning well, there are conditions where I could bleed to death. If I cut my finger, do I have to eat a healthy sandwich for it to heal? Do I have to take a nap? Jump on a treadmill? Funny, but do you see the difference? Those choices are good to help rebuild your house, but that is not where health comes from. Health is about function.

Remember our definition of health? A condition of wholeness in which all the organs are functioning 100% of the time. Our body is designed for *homeostasis*.

That's why people who do unhealthy things are still healthy; because their bodies don't get out of homeostasis. What's homeostasis?

The definition for homeostasis is very familiar in the chiropractic world:

> *A self-regulating process by which biological systems tend to maintain stability while adjusting conditions that are optimal for survival. If homeostasis is successful, life continues. If unsuccessful, disaster or death ensues. The stability attained is actually a dynamic equilibrium, in which continuous change occurs yet relatively uniform conditions prevail.*

Your body was built for normal function, and that is the best place for it to be.

Homeostasis is the scientific word, but all it really means is balance, or normal function. For some of you, this balance is simply between health and disease, but there is more to it. The body has three states: normal function, adaptation, and disease. There is ebb and flow within those states. Your body was built for normal function, and that is the best place for it to be. Oftentimes we spend a lot of time in the adaptation state before moving to the disease state. Nobody worries about the state they are in until they reach the disease state. They don't worry about it because their body is doing all the work.

Adaptation is the state between normal function and where symptoms show up. You can be in this state for a long time and not know it unless you're properly tested. You could wait until you've moved into the disease state; that's when we see those fires. Let's say your hormones are really high. Your body has left homeostasis and is in the adaptation state. If it stays there a long time, it will go to the disease state. The same happens if your hormones are really low. Your body is in the adaptation state; if it stays there long enough it will go into the disease state. That can be said for any situation that indicates your body has been knocked out of homeostasis.

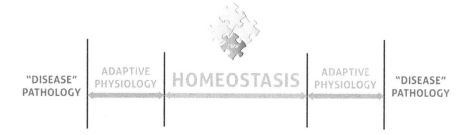

The reason why people are so sick today is because we jump back and forth between the states of adaptation and disease, never landing back in normal function. Our entire health care system reflects this. If your M.D. runs a test, they're going to be testing for disease and treating your symptoms. Your tests look fine until one day you show up and you have cancer. Then they treat your disease with a drug but you stay in dysfunction.

The only way to stop the cycle between adaptation and disease is to find out what is triggering the body and remove it so the body can return to balance or homeostasis.

One thing that sets The Wellness Way Approach apart is how we view the body as a collective whole. If you present one symptom, it may be reflective of a health challenge in a seemingly unrelated part of the body. However, we know there are no unrelated organs or systems within the body. Everything is connected like an intricate Swiss watch.

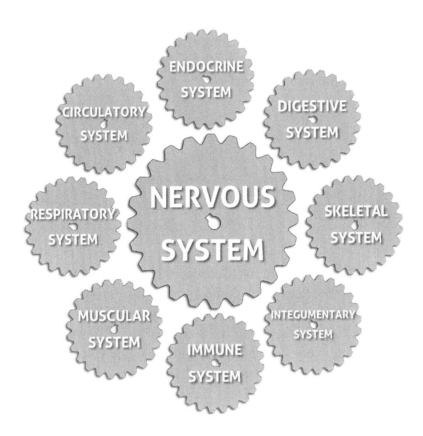

The Swiss Watch Principle:

If you take the back off of a Swiss watch, you see a bunch of gears. Some of them are large and some are small. Some move really fast while others move slowly. They all have a specific action they need to do for the time to keep properly. Imagine that the smallest or slowest gear stops working, or it breaks a tooth and doesn't work correctly. What happens? Well that's easy, right? It stops working or doesn't keep time accurately. Even the smallest gear affects how it keeps time. Each and every gear is needed.

The body is just like that. It is very complex and composed of many, many parts. Did you know your big toe controls your heart? Yes, really. If I smash your toe what happens to your heart rate? It goes up. Why? Because even that little gear can affect everything from your heart rate to your cholesterol. That's why it is important to not look at just one gear. If you have symptoms happening with your heart, they might be coming from one of the other gears. You can't just treat the heart with medication. It most likely could be a whole different gear that is making that symptom happen, and those medications have side effects.

Did you know your big toe controls your heart? Yes, really.

Has anyone ever taken a medication for heart issues and later discovered the medication damaged their liver? The human body is like a Swiss watch with many gears all working together in harmony. You cannot treat one system (gear) without affecting them all.

For example, detoxification is a very important gear; but it is only one gear. There are others, the gear of proper nutrition, the gear of chiropractic care, the gear of proper mental health (such as the proper handling of stress), and the gear of proper hormone function and so on. If you have even one gear not working properly, you cannot be healthy.

If a person receives regular chiropractic care but eats fast food all the time and handles his/her stress poorly, this person will not be able to achieve true and complete health. Likewise, if a person takes care of proper nutrition and proper detoxification but neglects the gear of proper care of the nervous system, he or she will never achieve complete health. We must have all the gears working together in harmony—this is complete health.

We address the cause (or causes) of ill health, not just the symptoms.

To sum up, it's important to look at each individual as unique. Clinically, we have to look at all the gears as a whole. That's why the medical or natural approach won't work. We have to find out what gear is being stressed and how. The gear can be the GI. As we know the GI can affect a lot of things; but so can the liver, the pancreas, the heart and many other gears. We look for which organ is being stressed to see how it could be causing a cascade of problems throughout the body. We look at the whole "watch" not just a part of it. We address the cause (or causes) of ill health, not just the symptoms.

You just learned about one of the core foundational principals I work from each day. When a patient comes in with depression, they have probably been working with doctors who scanned their brain and couldn't find a problem. Patients usually come to us after years of going to doctors and not finding the problem. Those doctors did what they could, but they didn't look at the hormones, the gut, or other systems in the body that could be causing this depression. They were looking at one gear. They needed to look at the whole watch.

Erin's Story

My family started seeing Dr. Patrick at The Wellness Way when two of our three daughters had adverse reactions to childhood vaccines.

Two years later, I noticed a lump in my breast. I was 32-years-old. The first thing I did was call The Wellness Way. I was able to see Dr. Patrick immediately. To say I was anxious is an understatement, but we found a fantastic community. When you walk in the door, you know you are in good hands. While I was meeting with Dr. Patrick, one of the front desk associates took two of my young daughters, so I could have a focused discussion. The first thing Dr. Patrick did was help me calm down. After an exam, he had me schedule an appointment with my OB/GYN to order a mammogram and ultrasound. He assured me he was confident I would be told the cyst was benign. He said they would watch it over the next several years. Dr. Patrick went on to ask a few more questions. By the time I left that first appointment, I felt much more confident.

The next appointment with my OB/GYN went as Dr. Patrick predicted. She did a quick breast exam, ordered the mammogram and ultrasound. During that time of waiting for appointments, our family had other visits with Dr. Patrick. Each time he would give me pieces of information to research. He already knew what I was going to face and wanted to prepare me. His confidence calmed me and my husband immeasurably.

Immediately after the mammogram, I was taken for additional testing. After a few days, I received a phone call. I was told the cyst was benign and they would keep an eye on it. I went back to Dr. Patrick armed with my good news. His answer was simple. I was "safe" for now, but my estrogen levels were abnormally high. I had a choice to make. I could either let things go and in 3-5 years I'd most likely be facing a cancer diagnosis with 3 young daughters and a husband in my mid-thirties. Or, I could work to get healthy now. It was an easy decision. Let's do this and get healthy! The date was October 17.

Dr. Patrick laid out the plan for me. I would have a very restricted diet for six months and the first few weeks would be especially intense. At the end of six months, I'd feel like a whole different woman. I was also excited at the prospect of losing the extra 40 pounds I was carrying. I had recently met a young woman about my age at church who had won her battle with breast cancer. I asked her what she knew about estrogen fed cysts and breast cancer. She pointed at her now flat chest and hair freshly grown back and told me she wished she had known more.

Remember that restricted diet and the date? The very next day was my daughter's birthday. I chose to give her a healthy momma and not have a piece of cake; and for the daughter who had a birthday two weeks later; and the next daughter, 3 days after the second. I said "no" to unhealthy eating at Thanksgiving, Christmas and all the holiday gatherings; including New Years, Valentine's Day, my husband's birthday and our wedding anniversary. Finally, six months later, on my birthday I was able to indulge in a piece of fruit. Dr. Patrick was and is right. Food is emotional. Your health is largely dictated by the eating choices you make.

I had a lot of questions from family and friends. I didn't want sympathy. I didn't need critics. This was an intentional decision to give my children a healthy mother, my husband a healthy wife and to reclaim my health. I cut out all sugar and nearly all my favorite foods. I learned a lesson that would affect many decisions we would make for health in the coming years. I was able to teach my beautiful daughters what has now become a family mantra – "food is fuel, not a friend". Was it hard? Yes! Was it worth it? Undoubtedly.

I've not been back to the OB/GYN for the last 10 ½ years. Why? The cyst dissolved, and had I followed their advice, I wouldn't be where I am today. My husband may have been a single father with three young daughters. I didn't want to play their guess and wait game. There was too much at stake.

For any woman wondering if taking care of herself and/or her hormones is worth it – absolutely. Look at your children, look at your husband. Get over the "hard" and do the hard and right thing. There's too much life to live. Choose to live it.

CHAPTER 4

Stressors

Chiropractors deal with stress. This puts them in a unique position to look at health differently. I learned that from the beginning of my adventure to Palmer Chiropractic College. Stress happens. It's how we deal with it that can make or break our health. I was finishing up my last semester at the University of Wisconsin–Green Bay and had sent my transcripts off to Palmer Chiropractic College where I'd be going to school in October. It was June, and there were just days left to final exams. I got a call from the admissions office.

They said I was missing a class. I said, "I'm not missing any classes. I have them all."

They said, "Oh wait, you have an exercise physiology class, but that doesn't count as a physiology class."

I said, "That was a level 300 physiology class and I was told that would be approved. I start there in October! I'm not going to wait another semester to start for a physiology class that I took." My mind and heart were racing.

They said, "Listen, we have a community college here that offers that course. You can finish it in six weeks. Then you can start school early." I had a choice to make either start in July or start in February. I asked when the class started. Monday! I'm a twenty-two-year-old guy in Green Bay, Wisconsin on Tuesday, with exams to finish. Class would start in Iowa on Monday, I didn't have much money, and I had nowhere to live. What did I do?

I scrambled. I finished my exams on Friday. I found a room to rent in a house with upper level chiropractic students. My parents and I packed up their pick up and headed to Iowa. I made it down there in time to take the course I needed.

I went home six weeks later to visit the weekend before I officially started at Palmer Chiropractic College and bad luck struck me again on my way back to Iowa. I was in Illinois, twenty miles from the Iowa border, when my car died. I couldn't get it started again, so I tried to flag someone down. No one would stop. Finally, this college kid heading to St. Ambrose University in the same town stops. He says he'll drive me to Ambrose, but I'll have to find a ride from there. I hopped in. When we got there, it was the middle of the night. There was no ride to be found, so I walked six miles to my new house with all that I could carry. I was stressed about how I was going to tow and fix my car, but I had class in the morning. Moral of the story? Stress is everywhere. We encounter it every day.

Some people say I'm just a chiropractor, but I'm proud of the potential of chiropractic. People say chiropractors are just pain doctors. I disagree. I'm proud of what I can do. Chiropractic helps me look at things differently. Through studying chiropractic, I learned what stresses are and how stress impacts the body.

What damages our health? What knocks our body out of homeostasis? Stress, or what we call the 3-T's in chiropractic.

Some people say I'm just a chiropractor, but I'm proud of the potential of chiropractic.

Traumas, toxins and thoughts damage our health. These are the 3-T's that chiropractic was meant to address at its foundation. Unfortunately, due to a wide variety of reasons, chiropractic has gotten away from its original directive. This means the value of what chiropractic can do is being overlooked. The 3-T's are the stresses that disrupt homeostasis. Stress is a stimulus that can produce mental or physiological reactions that may lead to illness. Technically speaking, stress is a disruption to homeostasis which may be triggered by alarming experiences.

Chiropractors are in the best position to help with physical stress or trauma. What does a chiropractor really do? Remove physical stress. You may be thinking, *no Doc, my chiropractor makes my pain go away.* Have you ever gotten adjusted and the pain did not go away? Let me raise my hand first. Have you ever gotten adjusted and your headache did not go away? Let me raise my hand first. Today we are so dominant in the fire department medical system; we define all professionals from that perspective. That's not true though. Chiropractors do just one thing. They are the carpenter doctor who removes that physical stress. But usually that's not the only stress. There are other stresses our bodies are exposed to because of our choices. If the body has a symptom, it is adapting to a stress. We can find out what that stress is and remove it.

To really understand how to keep the body in balance, we must understand each of the 3-T's.

What Is Trauma?

Anything that puts the body under physical stress.

If I run at you and attack you, what is going to happen to your heart rate? It goes up. What is going to happen to your blood sugar? It goes up. What happens to your cholesterol level? It goes up. Are you seeing a trend here? If we draw your blood at that moment what will medical

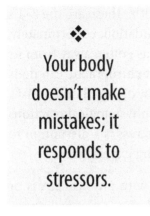

Your body doesn't make mistakes; it responds to stressors.

and natural doctors think? They will look at the results and say you are sick. What is your body really doing? It is responding to physical stress on your body. Your body doesn't make mistakes; it responds to stressors.

Remember that big toe example? If I smash your toe what happens to your heart rate? It goes up. Blood pressure? It goes up. Sugar? It goes up. Cholesterol? It goes up. That is a physical trauma. Your body will adapt to the physical trauma it encounters daily. No matter who you are, your body encounters trauma. Heck, your body encountered trauma coming into the world through your mama's birth canal. Don't try to tell me you don't have any physical trauma.

That's why when people say that they don't need to get adjusted, or their kid doesn't need to get adjusted, I respond, "wait…. you're telling me your child has no chance of physical trauma? Did your child learn to walk? Did they fall? Does she ever cross her legs? Does he ever lift things incorrectly?" See what I'm saying? When you remove that trauma, you leave room for the body to heal. All chiropractic really does is remove that physical trauma so the body can adapt. The body just wants to heal.

Let me give you another example. Let's say your plane was rerouted from Hawaii to Green Bay, Wisconsin during winter. You packed for summer, not the frigid temps of the frozen tundra. If you went outside in shorts and a tank top, you would be pretty cold. What would happen if you stayed out there in negative temperatures for a long time? Your body would send all the blood to your core to protect the vital organs. If you stayed out there long enough, could you lose your fingers and toes? Yes. That was an adaptation of the body. The body didn't make a mistake. It tried to adapt to the stressors, and kept you alive. It was your choice to walk outside and stay out there. The body always has to adapt, regardless of your choices. Your body always makes the right choices, even when you don't.

Speaking of choices, our modern, fast-paced, quick and easy lives mean we make a lot of choices that expose us to toxins.

What Are Toxins?

When I was a kid, my grandpa owned a bar across the street from our house. Every day, I would go across the street, open up the fridge, and grab a Coke. Then he'd give me a Kit Kat. To this day, I still want a Coke and a Kit Kat. No matter how healthy I eat, the memories associated with those foods make me want them still. I know now these are just one example of the many toxins our bodies encounter every day.

Toxin exposure begins in your mother's uterus. Her toxins became your toxins as they traveled through the placenta, and it didn't stop there. When you were born, you were most likely vaccinated and injected with toxins. The food you eat and even the water you drink can expose you to toxins even if you are eating really healthy. Toxins like lead in paint and toys, prescription drugs, beauty products, soaps, shampoos, and cleaning products. Toxins are inflammatory foods like sugar, dairy, and wheat. Even if you have reduced your exposure by being careful not to use toxic products, and eat super healthy foods, toxins are still in the air you breathe and water you drink.

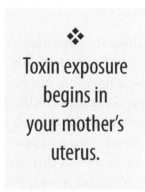

❖

Toxin exposure begins in your mother's uterus.

I know what you are thinking …*but Doc, our bodies naturally detoxify.* That's true, the body is built to detoxify. Our bodies can only handle so much before it becomes difficult for the body to naturally detoxify. Toxins build up when the detoxification mechanisms cannot keep up with the production of cellular wastes, or the absorption of toxins from the intestines. In other words, garbage is coming in at a faster rate than your body can process it and safely remove it. Those toxins build up and can make us very sick.

Exposure to xenoestrogens are very common in today's modern society. To make it simple, let's call this chemical, "estrogen". Xenoestrogens are a sub category of chemical endocrine disruptors that have an estrogen-like effect. What do you think it does to the body's homeostasis if you are throwing in a bunch of fake estrogen? These chemicals are everywhere. BPA, phthalates and parabens are common xenoestrogens. They are in plastics, household cleaning products, dryer sheets, cookware, food and beauty products. These are products people come in contact with every day, and they are building up in the body of a high percentage of people.

There are some toxins that knock some people right out of homeostasis. Mold can be toxic for many people. It is a hidden killer that can cause inflammation, hormone imbalance, and immunity issues. In chronic exposure it can be hard to identify. The toxicity suppresses the immune system which can trigger other illnesses. And since finding the source often means relocation if they find that their home is the source, many are unable to eliminate the source or can't afford to. In reality, they can't afford not to. People look at their symptoms and the illness and don't always connect them to mold sickness. In the long term, this can lead to even more serious illness like cancer or autoimmune disorders.

Most people don't see the toxins because the effect doesn't seem immediate. The body has to respond to all of your choices.

If I give you a shot of gasoline to drink, what happens to your blood pressure? It's going to go up. You are probably going to puke, run a fever, and get diarrhea. Your body is adapting to the toxin. You're not sick. Your body is trying to adapt. It's trying to bring everything back to homeostasis. You may have been the one who made the bad choice to drink the gasoline, but your body is making positive choices so it can adapt.

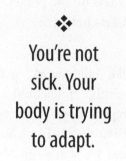

You're not sick. Your body is trying to adapt.

All illness is a long-term adaptation for survival. We look at things that stress the body and go from there. When we assess a patient, we look for what is stressing the body. Imagine if I stressed you out like crazy and then you went for a check-up at the medical doctor right after. They are going to look at you and tell you, "your blood pressure is high. Let's inhibit and stimulate the body to a normal level." They'll use drug or surgery intervention. What an incomplete way of looking at it! They never looked at what was causing the high blood pressure in the first place. Wouldn't it make more sense to look at what is triggering the stress and remove that?

That's why understanding toxins and detoxification is so important. We will talk about that more later. There's another "T" that we have to discuss and this one is a big one in today's society.

What Are Thoughts?

This is the stress most people think about when they think of stresses! It's the mental stress that I encountered when I started chiropractic school. It's your mental stress that you encounter every day. It's huge! Most people don't realize the impact it makes. Now, don't get stressed out about your stress just yet. First, let's start with who stresses out more, men or women? Women. Who causes women the most stress? This is where the audience laughs, and calls out "Men!" Guess what—they're right! I'll prove it to you that men are one of the biggest contributors to illness on the planet today. I'm not joking! Hang with me though guys, it gets better.

Every day we are bombarded with worries like bills, work, getting kids to school, health, household chores, and all the expectations to keep all these things afloat. Then we find out how bad stress is for us and we stress out about that. That means we are up at night stressing about our stress. It's a never-ending cycle!

It's important to reduce stress because it can impact every system in your body, and when one system gets out of whack so can others. For example, when stress puts our body into the fight or flight mode it can impact our digestive system, and your body won't be able to digest the food you ate. This can lead to acid reflux, colon problems, hormone problems, high blood pressure, and so much more.

❖
We are up at night stressing about our stress. It's a never-ending cycle!

Christy's Thoughts

That pivotal day that Patrick found me—you see, I get it now. When Patrick told me, "don't worry, you will be okay," he was removing one of my stressors without me realizing it. He knew that I was depleting my hormones worrying about my health and future. So, when I hear friends or some of our patients frustrated about the length of time that the healing process takes, I just need to say that I UNDERSTAND! My biggest piece of advice: Trust the process! You, as a patient, need to step back, follow the guidance of a Wellness Way doctor, and stop stressing yourself out! All you are doing is prolonging your healing process. I did not get well overnight. It took many years of continuous baby steps in the right direction and Patrick asking different

> *questions in order to come up with different solutions to what I was going through.*

Mental stress can make you very sick, especially if you are a woman. It is the biggest reason I see patients in my clinic. Mental stress can really impact a woman's health starting with her hormones. I want you to think about this. You can get adjusted, pull all the chemicals out of your body and eat organic but guess what is ten times more disruptive to health than anything else. Mental stress. It will kill you. All doctors are taught this. So, back to my study. I started to study women. I studied why they stressed out so much. I polled women eighteen years ago and I still ask them today. What do women care about? EVERYTHING. But what are the top three things that cause the most stress?

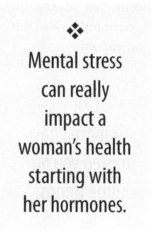

❖
Mental stress can really impact a woman's health starting with her hormones.

WOMEN	MEN
1. Men	1. Work
2. Children	2. Sex
3. Weight	3. Kids

Here's where I may surprise some women. Women, it's very clear where we are on your stress list. Ladies, where are you on our stress list? You're not. There's only one way you can stress out a guy, ladies. I'm going to show you there's a biological reason why in a few chapters if you will be patient with me. The rewards for your health and relationships will be worth it!

Some people might call these men disgusting, perverted pigs. I disagree, and if you stick with me, for the next few chapters you will find out why there is this biological difference that comes down to hormones. Stresses impact all of us. Understanding the 3-T's helps us understand how to mitigate that stress so that we can find and maintain homeostasis.

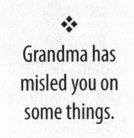

❖

Grandma has misled you on some things.

Most of us know common stressors to our bodies. That's when people get caught up in the idea of moderation. People say everything's okay in moderation. I disagree. Most grandmas are a fan of moderation. You can also swap out for mom, dad, aunt, uncle or any other person who has helped shape the way you approach food including grandpas who give you a Coke and a Kit Kat bar just for crossing the street. Grandma has misled you on some things. You may be thinking, *Doc, are you saying my grandma was wrong?* Well, grandmas are right about a lot of things—and we love them dearly—but in their quest to indulge us, they encourage some unhealthy habits.

Let me explain. Grandma comes to you after you've started to eat healthy. She brings a plate of chocolate chip cookies with all the unhealthy, highly processed ingredients and she sweetly says, "Here honey, I have some cookies for you," and you say, "No thank you, Grandma, I'm not going to eat those." And Grandma says, "Everything is good in moderation!" Grandma loves you, but her perspective is wrong. I disagree with moderation. Your body doesn't know if something is good or not. It knows if something is inflammatory and creates stress or if it is not inflammatory. It doesn't know moderation. It doesn't stop the inflammation process just because you only eat that food once in a while.

Eating is one of the most emotional things we do. Let me give you an example. Let's say I gave some health advice to a married couple; don't have sex for a week. Now the guy will be kinda mad, the gal will be just fine. Right? But here's another angle. If I tell that same couple to fast for three days, they'll both hate me. Food carries a lot of emotional influence. Just to help understand this point, I've defined moderation for us:

> *Moderation is your emotional justification to eat something bad for you.*

It's just emotional, that's all it is. In the end it all boils down to your choices.

Your body responds to your choices, regardless if they are good or not. So, you say, "Oh come on, it's just one cookie!" But the body still has to do what? Adapt to your choices. Is not getting a regular chiropractic adjustment a bad habit? Yes, it is, so your body is going to adapt to not getting adjusted. If you eat a bunch of processed sugar cookies, your body adapts. If you are mentally stressing out about your in-laws visiting, your body has to adapt to it. Picture yourself getting away from people stressing you out, and locking yourself in a room for an hour. What happens to your blood pressure? It goes back to normal. Blood sugar? It goes back to normal. Cholesterol? It goes back to normal. What stresses out the body? Trauma, toxins and thoughts. Your body will respond to those. Your body will adapt to those.

That's how disease happens. Do we respond to the symptoms or do we respond to the triggers? It seems pretty simple to me. Where it gets a little more complicated is that there is usually more than one stressor and people respond to triggers uniquely. This is

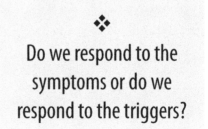

❖

Do we respond to the symptoms or do we respond to the triggers?

especially true if we are looking at the differences between a man and a woman. In this politically correct world, we don't talk about stresses the way they need to be talked about. Men and women are different. Yes, men and women need to be valued equally; however, in that argument we must understand that valuing them equally does not mean they are *the same*. We need to be able to appreciate and empower both, along with their biological differences. For our health and our relationships, this is absolutely necessary.

CHAPTER 5

Don't Kill the Messenger

Men and women are different. That doesn't mean one is of less value than the other. It just means they are biologically different. I understand how women are biologically made. I don't try to make them something they're not, and I hope the women in my life don't try to make me into something I'm not. It would be a difficult task though—my testosterone is high, which makes me confident in who I am. You'll learn more about how this works later. For now, we need to understand that it is not only okay, but necessary for women and men to be recognized as different.

We live in a time when everybody is saying we (men and women) are the same. I'm going in the exact opposite direction. I disagree! It's not because I'm a male or a chauvinist; it's because what they are saying doesn't make any sense. It doesn't make any clinical sense. When it comes down to it, we are confusing people. We are treating them all the same and it's leading to sickness. All these women are coming in sick as can be, and it's the same for the guys. Everyone is sick. Why? Because they don't understand who they are or how they are biologically made. We got away from understanding the differences between the genders somewhere in the midst of trying to make them equal.

Now for those ladies who are getting uncomfortable about this, please, let's slow down a bit and hear me out. I never once said you are weaker.

You can have a baby. I can't. You're nurturing. I'm not. You dominate in a lot of things that guys can't. Equality can't happen simply because we're not *equal*. However, valuing each other for our individual gifts and what we can bring to the table **is** possible. We can't be like you and you can't be like us. Here's an example: if a woman has a sex drive like a man, she is going to end up with cancer. Why? Because that woman has high testosterone, which *isn't* normal for a woman. If a woman has a sex drive every day, then clinically I'm out of my mind worried about her. I want to get her tested to find out what is triggering her hormones out of balance. It's a signal that she has PCOS or some testosterone dominant hormone going on that will leave her very sick and potentially with cancer. It's biologically impossible for a lady to be healthy *and* masculine, the hormones simply don't allow it.

Have you ever seen little boys and girls play together? They get along just fine. Their hormones are quite similar and consistent. Then, that magical time called puberty comes about and turns the whole relationship upside down. They don't know if they love each other or hate each other. Throwing two cats in a burlap sack would be more peaceful than watching two pubescent adolescents of the opposite sex try to interact. What happened? They still have the same genes and phenotypes, but something has changed, and it's changed dramatically. Their hormones have started to change their childhood bodies into the bodies of a man and a woman. They may not be able to describe or explain it, but they can sure feel it—and so can everyone else around them.

> ❖
> **Have you ever seen little boys and girls play together? They get along just fine.**

We have gotten away from the biology-the actual science that in any other debate would be looked at as gospel. Today's culture has the idea that men and women are the same. Biologically, I will prove to you beyond a scientific doubt, there is *no way* a man and woman can think the same. Of course they can agree, but that's not what we're talking about. I'm saying they aren't actually thinking the same way. It's virtually impossible. It's physically impossible! There is just no way. There is no way my wife and I could think the same. Do you want to know why? Because we are biologically different. Here, I can prove it to you guys. Let's say I inject your wife with synthetic hormones. I guarantee within a week she will think differently. Do you know why? Because it will alter her brain. The same thing if we take a guy and inject him with a ton of testosterone. He's going to think differently very shortly. Do you want to know why? Lots of testosterone is going to affect his brain also. Ladies, you know this. Your hormones change throughout the month. Your mental pattern changes throughout the month. It's a **good** thing for a normal functioning body. Don't feel bad about it. It is what your body was born to do! Men's and women's hormones aren't designed to make us operate the same. Hormones are what make us who we are. It's what makes a man a man and a woman a woman. We are so dramatically, biologically different, but we are trying to force men to be women and women to be men. And now, as a result, we are seeing consequences in their health.

❖

Maybe, just maybe, men and women need to understand why they are different.

What's tragic is that this goes beyond health and impacts our relationships. There are two things I see all over the country: very sick women (and men too) and very disappointed women. Whether we realize it or not, our health can play a significant role in our relationships. Divorce is on the rise, and so is cancer, depression, and chronic illness. Could there be a reason or correlation? Maybe, just maybe, men and women need to understand why they are different.

I started speaking about this all from the physical aspect; but it became so much more when I heard from people whose health was improving. Women would say, "Hey Doc, I'm psychologically better and more in love with my husband, my marriage is so much better." Men would come up to me all excited, "I have a better sex drive and energy levels. My marriage is better!" That's how my Hormone Connection seminar got started.

As patients started to see healthy results, they also had really positive side effects. How incredible is that? Marriages were being saved! When I started to get them physically healthy, their mentality changed, which resulted in their relationships getting better. As soon as you learn this information, it changes your thinking. Once you change your thinking, we are ten steps closer to changing your health.

> ❖
> **Once you change your thinking, we are ten steps closer to changing your health.**

One night after a seminar, a man came up to me and said, "I wish I would have known this forty years ago. I would have treated my wife differently." That's huge! When both men and women understand the concepts I teach, a relationship can change direction. Here's the key: You have to understand how hormones work. They will dictate the physical and mental aspects of the body. Don't believe me? Keep reading and let me prove it to you!

Even though we highly recommend bringing your spouse to the Hormone Connection seminar, one of the most frequent comments I always hear from women after a seminar is, "I wish my husband would have been here to hear this too!" When both spouses are on the same page it makes caring for their health so much easier. When a patient comes into my office, I prefer to meet with couples. It makes the most sense. When both partners hear the message from the same source, there will be less confusion and we will be able to communicate more clearly. Also, it will help the person we are most focusing on to have a support person. Often there are real and practical steps the support person can do to help our patient. That's why I've written this book as if I'm speaking to both men and women even though I know that women make approximately 95% of the healthcare decisions.

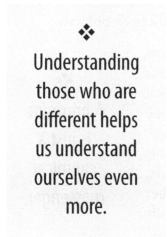

Understanding those who are different helps us understand ourselves even more.

If the wife gets this approach and she shares it with her husband, they will start an amazing process of getting healthy and having a happier marriage together. But wait—I'm not excluding you singles out there. This book is still for you! You can learn more about yourself and learn about others too. It's handy to know about both genders in work and life. Understanding those who are different helps us understand ourselves even more. After all, knowing someone and understanding someone are two totally different things.

So, let's start breaking this down. In my seminars, I often ask women what they want in a man. I hear things like:

Compassionate, kind, a good listener, thoughtful, gentle

Ladies, I think I may have found the problem. You aren't looking for a man, what you just described is another woman! When you understand the basic biological differences in our hormones, you understand the simple fact remains that men and women are very different to their core. No matter what media and Hollywood would have us think today, we aren't the same, and it has little to do with the clothes we prefer to wear. A man can't be a woman and a woman can't be a man. There will be so much less confusion in this world once we get over the notion of "gender confusion."

Remember when I talked about how easy it was for kids to play together before puberty? That's because at that time their hormone levels are roughly the same. So, let's say a child hits puberty and their gender-specific hormones haven't 'kicked in', resulting in what some label 'gender confusion'—this means they are SICK! They aren't an opposite gender trapped in the wrong body; their hormones are way off and not communicating with the rest of the body properly.

To understand the difference between the sexes we must understand hormones. What is a hormone? It's a group of specialized chemical messengers that make up the whole endocrine system. Each hormone has a special message. A hormone doesn't really do anything on its own. It's released by a gland like the pituitary, ovary or testicle. That hormone goes to another cell and tells it what to do. But it doesn't really do anything other than act as a communicator. Then it breaks down and gets reabsorbed. A hormone is just a chemical messenger. When

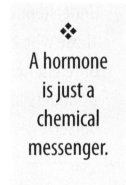

A hormone is just a chemical messenger.

people say, "I'm crabby. My hormones are off." What does that mean? It means the messenger is off. You know that saying, "Don't blame the messenger?"

Don't blame the messenger if something is off in your body. It's not the messenger's fault that something is triggering stress in your body. It's just telling the body the message it was given by the glands as to how the body can adapt. If the adrenals are stressed, that will impact the messenger. This can happen in all areas of your body impacting various messengers that help the different systems of the body function. Everything from digestion to reproduction or thinking to growth.

Men and women have different glands and different messengers. Don't blame me for biology! I'm just the messenger here. This isn't my opinion. It's the physiological makeup of males and females. We need to really get into hormones to understand how they make us different. Since guys are the simplest, we are going to talk about how they work first. Once we figure out men, it will be a lot easier to understand women. You thought it was hard? This guy figured it out, and if I can, so can you! So, what makes a guy work? Keep reading.

CHAPTER 6

Why is He so Confident?

Why am I so confident? Because I have made sure the primary source of my testosterone is optimized and fully functioning! I'm talking about testicles. 95-97% of testosterone production happens there. The other 3% happens in the adrenals. Testosterone is what makes a man who he is, but there is so much that goes into it. Once you understand the body is like a Swiss watch, you understand that you can't just add testosterone to make a man. If a man has low testosterone, it's not that he is getting old or that his testicles aren't working. Let me show you how testosterone is made. It will help explain a lot. You'll understand why men have the traits that make them men and confident about it.

Testosterone is what makes a man who he is, but there is so much that goes into it.

It all starts in the brain. You'll learn later how to master the guy's brain. The pituitary gland, or what we call the "master gland," is a little gland that hangs in the brain. This is where our story of testosterone production starts. The things that happen in the brain can have an effect on testosterone production or any hormone production. The first thing you have to have is luteinizing hormone. The pituitary gland gets a lot of feedback from the hypothalamus. The hypothalamus will release a gonadotropin releasing hormone that tells the pituitary to create follicle stimulating hormone (FSH) and luteinizing hormone (LH). LH is the big producer of testosterone. LH is the hormone that goes down to the testicle and binds to a cell. If LH isn't normal you can't have testosterone. It starts in the pituitary; that's why it's called the master gland. LH travels in the bloodstream down to the testicle.

Remember, this is where the half mile of tubules are that are misleadingly called balls. The testicle is actually a casing. It's a bunch of tubules, a bunch of cells put together. Some of those cells are Leydig cells. Those Leydig cells have little receptors; those receptors are looking for LH hormone. Those Leydig cells need LH to be stimulated to work. That's the first part of testosterone production.

What you need next is LDL, or cholesterol. I know most of you are probably thinking, *LDL is bad!* No! It's not bad. It's needed by the body for homeostasis. We will talk more about that later. The only thing you need to start the production of testosterone is LH and LDL (LDL is produced by the liver). What we know about the body is that it operates like a Swiss watch. What's happening in the brain and the liver can impact testosterone. The liver converts hormones and regulates the balance of your sex hormones. If something is off in the brain or the liver, your hormones can be way off. It's not just the testicle. The body is a combination of massive moving parts. To think everything has to do with just the testicle is incorrect. You can't just add testosterone and fix everything. Anything that disrupts the brain, or the hypothalamus, can disrupt LH production which can disrupt testosterone production.

Testosterone is responsible for the physical and mental differences between men and women. It gives us energy, it gives us muscle development, and it gives us our sexual drive. Hormones also change us mentally. Testosterone gives a man great confidence. Every healthy man, regardless of his age, thinks he's amazing. Right, ladies? Do you ever see your husband in front of a mirror? He's flexing and checkin' himself out. It doesn't matter how old he is. Testosterone gives us this great confidence! Ladies, you don't have the amount of testosterone we do so you tend to down play it. When a man can be confident and unashamed, that's healthy. Don't put him down for his confidence – encourage that boy! That's normal and healthy. The second function of testosterone is to keep him motivated and driven. Testosterone is why he does what he does; it is a very driving hormone. If somebody were to break into your house tonight, which of you will get up to chase the criminal? Your man will, why? Because when testosterone rises, it makes him aggressive. Ladies, you like that; until you create the same reaction in him as if a criminal who broke into your

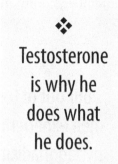

Testosterone is why he does what he does.

house. Yikes! Remember the big steroid hormone craze of the 80's? It was a craze alright. What happens when you give a man a synthetic testosterone to supplement his natural testosterone? He will go crazy with aggression.

Think about it. Who commits the most violent crimes, men or women? There isn't even a comparison. Does that mean you should hate men? No, men commit three times as many violent crimes as women. I don't intend to create an argument—those are the facts. With that fact in mind, does it mean police hate men? No, it does not mean police are targeting men. Why then are men committing more violent crimes? By nature, men are more aggressive; that's why they commit more violent crimes. If the testosterone gets too high from steroids or a tumor, it can cause them to commit a violent crime. It's one of the side effects of steroid drugs. The testosterone range for women is between five and forty Ng/dL. Guy's range is between 350-1200 Ng/dL. Even at the lowest end, a guy is more than seven times higher than the testosterone at the highest end of the range for a woman. A man's always going to be more aggressive than a woman. This idea that we can be mentally or biologically the same is not true.

Now some of you might have examples of men who don't have high confidence or motivation. These stories are all too common. But remember, common does not mean normal.

Four out of ten men experience hypogonadism, which is another name for low testosterone.

"Doc, my husband sits on the couch a lot more lately, but overall he's a healthy guy," says a woman in the office, there to take care of her hormonal health. My response? Oh no he's not healthy! You know what her other complaint was? He isn't interested in sex. Does that sound healthy to you? It sounds like he has low testosterone to me. Ladies, if your husband isn't chasing you around every day, it's a sign he's sick. Before that sign happens, you may notice he loses his spark to get stuff done. This guy is not alone. Four out of ten men experience hypogonadism, which is another name for low testosterone. Despite what the medical community has told you, low testosterone is not a natural part of aging. Remember, common is not normal.

This woman was sitting in my office because her hormones were off, but she didn't notice the signs that there was something wrong with her husband's main hormone. When women have symptoms of imbalanced hormones, they know what's causing it. They might think there is nothing they can do about it, but they know what is to blame. When a man's main hormone is off, there are mental factors that many will just brush off.

Most men don't get their testosterone tested until they are older and experiencing physical symptoms. The majority of testosterone is produced in the testicles for men and it stimulates male characteristics. It can impact a man's health, sperm production, bone mass, muscle mass, sex drive, energy, facial hair, self-confidence and more. Low testosterone can lead to major health problems including cancer. We want it to be at good levels.

What people don't know is most men will experience more mental problems before the physical problems manifest. Let me say that again. Men will go through more mental changes than physical changes when their testosterone comes down. So, when you see your man getting lazy and demotivated it's an early sign something is going wrong.

How is it going wrong? In rare cases it can be a tumor, but most of the time it is because of unhealthy habits. If a young man has unhealthy habits as he ages, his testosterone will go down. It's not because he's aging! It's because of his unhealthy habits, including all the sugar he may be eating.

You need to get your man tested. Low testosterone is not normal. Just like PMS is not normal, menopause symptoms are not normal, endometriosis is not normal, or any of the other hormonal conditions that we relate to women. It's one of my most popular quotes for a reason… common is not normal. Women and men need to take care of their hormonal balance. Men and women are different, so their hormones are different. But whether it's a man or a woman, if their hormones are off, they will end up very sick.

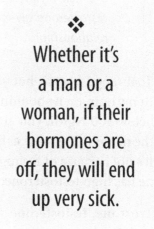

❖
Whether it's a man or a woman, if their hormones are off, they will end up very sick.

We dismiss it as aging, but it is a real sign of testosterone levels that are going down. It's not normal for an aging man to have their testosterone go down. Clinically, all of our clinics could show you men in their eighties who have high testosterone. Testosterone levels are independent of age. Ask my wife. You can ask a healthy male. Ask a woman who has a healthy male. You know what they say about the healthy male? That boy is always going. My wife will tell you that I'm a healthy male!

CHRISTY'S THOUGHTS

> *Yes, no doubt about it—my husband is a healthy male! It's the confidence and boldness that attracted me to him in the first place. I admit that early in our dating and marriage I didn't understand some of those masculine traits, but now I do and have come to embrace them in my husband. I don't want to change him. Testosterone traits define a man. God molds and defines his character. I am very aware of men that I encounter who are very obviously sick and don't even realize it, sadly, until their marriages begin to fall apart. Ladies, get the men in your life tested!! Learn to love the God-given qualities that testosterone gives a man, your man, and you will transform your relationship!*

That range is wide, but you want to see good, high testosterone levels. In my opinion it shouldn't go below 500 Ng/dL. Man, if you're pushing below 500 Ng/dL you are going to have one demotivated boy. One of the major things to watch for ladies, is if your boy is starting to get lazy. It's not because of feelings. Testosterone is not impacted by feelings. If he has high testosterone, he is going to be on the move.

Trust me, testosterone will make the body do things. Don't believe me? Look under the covers in the morning. If your boy has high testosterone you will see evidence of the testosterone salute. Testosterone is highest in the morning and fluctuates throughout the day. Morning erections exist regardless of how a man feels. Don't make your man feel badly about this– that's a sign of a healthy boy! His normal physiology will make him get an erection in the morning. Why? As those testosterone levels come up…so does he. It's independent of how he feels. That's why when he gets demotivated you need to get that man's hormones checked.

Ladies, you are attracted to a strong, motivated man. You don't like a wimpy, demotivated man. Guys know this! That's why testosterone is so important to a man. This aggressive hormone makes us who we are. This is how biochemistry works. You want a feminized man? Let his testosterone come down. But you don't want that—it's not a good thing. When a guy sees himself, or women see the men in their lives (husbands, sons, fathers) becoming demotivated, it's time to make some changes with a new approach to how we see and appreciate guys.

CHAPTER 7

Men Are Simple

"Doc, my relationship with my husband has gotten so much better. The spark is back in our marriage!" I have heard this so many times, especially when I first started out in practice. I didn't start out talking about hormones and relationships. I started out talking about how to heal the body. What my patients and I found out was that being healthy improves relationships. Understanding the hormones improves relationships. I was just a doctor trying to give my patients the best functioning version of themselves. Better relationships was a happy side effect.

Here's one piece of relationship advice you can both thank me for. Imagine you've just had what I like to call a *passionate conversation*, some may call it a fight. Ladies, your hormones make you want to talk. Don't talk to him. His testosterone is too high; leave him alone. He'll cool off and come back with a much more level head and be able to have the conversation you want to have. Many devastating and mean things are said by husbands when they are mad. When he relaxes, that testosterone returns to normal and you are both able to speak calmly, he always says "honey, I didn't mean it that way." And he

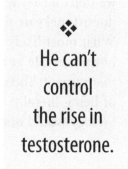

He can't control the rise in testosterone.

didn't. He was responding to the rise in testosterone due to the rise in tensions in the situation. He can't control the rise in testosterone. I'm not saying he shouldn't control his response—he absolutely should— but when people understand testosterone, they can have much more success during conflict. When his testosterone rises, it tells him to attack whatever is sitting in front of him. If that's you, it's a bad day. In no way am I justifying the horrific domestic abuse caused by disgusting men who are out of control. I'm explaining what a rapid rise of testosterone does in the brain.

Testosterone also makes him very single-task focused. Once you realize where it comes from, it's very obvious to see in various ways throughout his life. Ladies, your guy can only think about one thing at a time. Consider how quickly guys tend to climb any ladder of success. Men are driven because they can focus on just one thing at a time. Testosterone tells the guy's brain to go after whatever he sees. Think about that fact in terms of relationships. Ladies, do you think testosterone tells a guy:

"be nice to the girl"

"romance the girl"

"get her flowers"

NO! It tells him to "chase the girl!" See, you want us to be like you. But we don't have the same hormones you do, so we can't be like you. It doesn't make us any better or worse than you, it simply makes us men. What most likely attracted you to that guy was the opposite of your hormones. He pursued you with a clear purpose and was relentless in that pursuit. Today, politically, we think men and women are capable of being literally the same. They are not. They never could be; their biology would never allow it to happen.

In the evening, a man's testosterone starts to decrease a little bit. His ability to listen and focus increases. He's also more agreeable, passive and low key. Ladies, let me tell you step one in how to win with your man. If you try to tell your husband to do something in the morning—you might as well have not told him at all. Let me give you an example.

You ask him to take out the garbage. He's laser focused on the day ahead of him. He's not really listening to you and he leaves. When he closes the door and walks out, the garbage is still left there. Upset that he didn't listen and help, you begin to stress. During the day you imagine all the possible reasons why he didn't take out the garbage. We've all been there. On his side, he's forgotten about it the minute he left the door! Testosterone has him so focused he's in his own world. He simply didn't hear you, but you stew all day, either mad or with hurt feelings. You end up creating a lot of stress and can even make yourself sick due to the imaginary reasons you've created in your mind. When he comes home, he has been laser-focused, energetic and aggressive

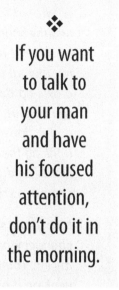

If you want to talk to your man and have his focused attention, don't do it in the morning.

all day and you've been imagining things and frustrated all day. Your first response is to question about why he didn't take out the garbage like you so sweetly asked him that morning. His response, "You didn't ask!" and you're off to the races with another fight. Ladies, understand, if you want to talk to your man and have his focused attention, don't do it in the morning. This will save so many fights. If his testosterone is normal, he's already in high gear and not hearing you. I know some call this selective hearing. He's really not trying to ignore you; his brain is just focused with the morning dose of testosterone he naturally needs to make it through the day.

CHRISTY'S THOUGHTS

I'm going to be honest, real and vulnerable with you. I made plenty of mistakes early in our marriage due to not understanding what testosterone did and how to keep my man healthy. No one teaches you about hormones or how our bodies are supposed to work and act, so how are we supposed to know what to do when things start to go wrong? To top that off, most people have never learned how to set healthy boundaries either. As I walked my rocky journey of becoming healthier, I realized that as my physical health began to improve, my mental health needed to change too. You see, when a person grows up dealing with constant health issues, a 'victim mentality' can emerge, and, when I realized that some of my words, thoughts and actions were not healthy, I had a choice to make. I could keep thinking the same old thoughts, speaking the same old destructive words, and doing the same old bad emotional habits, or I could choose to THINK DIFFERENTLY.

I chose and still choose to this day to examine myself daily and make changes when I see they don't line up with the priorities I have set in my life. Think of it this way—if you have a pebble in your shoe and walk on it all day long, what is your mood like? Probably irritable and perhaps over reactive, right? Well, if you remove the pebble, but don't address how you react to things, you may unintentionally be hurting others with the way you speak or respond to them. So, as you are healing physically, don't forget to take the time to do the 'hard-stuff' of getting brutally honest with yourself and healing emotionally as well.

The Man Zone

We've discussed the fact testosterone rises drastically during puberty and remains high his whole life. I want your man in the Man Zone all the time, that's normal.

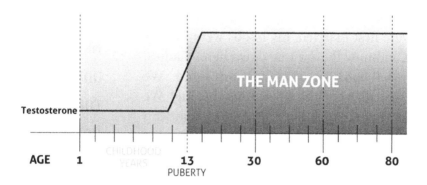

What do you think is the most common challenge with men in the Man Zone? I hear ladies whine, "But Doc, you don't understand, my husband wants sex every day!" My response is simple "that's a good, healthy boy!" Are guys perverted? Are they disgusting? Nope, sexually driven? Yes. And guess what. Men, that's part of being a man. Be proud of it! Women, you married him because you wanted a man. That's part of the package. Now remember, just because he wants it every day doesn't mean he gets it. A woman always has a choice and men have to do their homework. I do want those guys to stay in the Man Zone. If they don't, they'll get very sick. I'm going to teach you ladies how to build his testosterone and keep your man healthy. You can help him increase his testosterone, so you can get him to do virtually anything you want. I'm going to give you a To Do List. Don't worry, I'm not putting all the work on you. You get off easy. The men will have two To Do Lists. Trust me, they can handle it. They have testosterone to motivate them.

#1 Show the Boy

Let me explain this a bit. Ladies, men are visual creatures. They like seeing what they're chasing. Your favorite fluffy jammies that keep you toasty head to toe are not helping your cause in this instance. Think about it for a minute. Your coziest things are very likely not sexy. We love to pursue what we can see! I can already hear the arguments, "Doc, when we were first married, my boobs were way up here, and now they're way down here." Ladies, let me tell you something; we don't mind. We will hold them right where they belong! We will, we're nice like that. The only person who cares is you. We're big picture thinkers—we're into you, not the details! Most of the time we are completely unaware of the details. You know that. It's true in a number of areas in our lives, and it works here too. Let me share a story to illustrate this point.

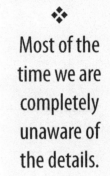

❖

Most of the time we are completely unaware of the details.

When I turned sixteen, I bought my first car for $150. It was a royal blue 1978 Pinto station wagon with no muffler. It was a chick magnet. I used to pull up to Crivitz High School and lean up next to my car like James Dean without the cigarette. I was so proud. You know why? Because it was mine. Ladies, that's the way a healthy man thinks about you. Just ask any man if he wants to see his wife in bed tonight. If he's a healthy boy and a real man, you know he will. He doesn't see the stretch marks, the extra few pounds and the sag you do. He sees his wife, and he's dang proud of her. That should reduce a lot of emotional stress for you ladies. If you know how this works, you can get him to do whatever you want—and you'll both be happier!

CHRISTY'S THOUGHTS

Ladies, this is so important and so SIMPLE to do…and if you value your man and your marriage this tip will become a fun, playful habit that you will share 'till death do you part! I guarantee that your man has some favorite 'spot' on your body, and no I'm not talking about 'the Man-Cave'! I'm talking about that 'special spot' on your body that, when he gets a glimpse of it, drives him crazy! And ladies, it's usually a spot on your body like the nape of your neck, small of your back, or other spot that is not considered 'private'. So, use it!!! Patrick's favorite 'spot' of mine is so easy for me to just enter a room and show him purposefully—and what's the purpose? He will have ME on his mind ALL DAY LONG! When he travels this has him missing me and wanting to rush home to me as well. Ladies, it is so important to be playful with your spouse. It's healthy and the kids don't even realize it's happening…they just see your healthy relationship.

#2 TALK TO THE BOY

You may think you talk to him all the time. But you talk to him in a way that feeds your hormones. Right now, we are talking about his hormones. There is a way you can talk to your man to get him to do what you want him to do all day. All you have to do tomorrow morning is grab that testosterone filled boy before he leaves for work and whisper into his ear, "Honey, tonight is going to be a good night!" What do you think your husband will be thinking about ALL DAY LONG? When he gets home, he's going to get the kids ready for bed, and do the dishes. He's going to do everything he needs to do because his testosterone has been stimulated to. You have a motivated man. That's how a man works. If you don't want to do that, the sad reality is, some other woman will. If you don't talk to him the way he needs to be talked to and you don't show him what he needs to see, some other girl will. It won't be intentional on his part. He'll be at work someday and when that pretty girl walks by and says something to him or dresses in a way that shows him a little more than he sees at home, he can't help but be stimulated. No, it's not a happy thought, but either you accept how this works, or you can be just as unhappy as the majority of marriages are today. We get wrapped up in the thought that men and women are created the same. They are not. Has the divorce rate in the last twenty years increased or decreased? That seems to be about the timing as to when we started trying to force men to be more like women. They are what they are. When we accept that men and women were created a specific, and different way, we'll all be able to get along much better. I know I keep hammering this point, but so does the media and our culture. Once we accept reality, we'll be able to move on from this. Until then, we'll have to continue to hammer this point over and over.

#3 Don't Feed the Boy

I know men like #1 and #2 but they're not going to like #3. As your husband gains too much weight, his testosterone will convert to another type of hormone, estrogens. That's why breast cancer is second to prostate cancer in men today. As their man boobs and the rest of them get larger, their hormones convert to estrogens. Fat does a very good job of producing and storing estrogens making those men become more female like in hormones.

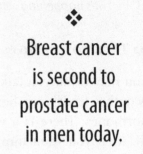

Breast cancer is second to prostate cancer in men today.

Estrogens rising too high are currently the only known cause of breast cancer. A few times after taking a man's blood work, I have had him fast for seventy-two hours and his testosterone would rise anywhere from 25-40%. Men need to cut the sugar, and men need to fast. I like to recommend a seventy-two-hour fast every three months to help with testosterone levels. Ladies, sometimes you may have to put the kibosh on him and tell him he needs to take a break for a couple of days. Remember how I told you about foods and emotions? It's just as true for guys as it is for women.

#4 Capture the Boy's Mind

My wife is a genius at this. I travel a lot. Sometimes she goes with me, but sometimes she doesn't and I'm by myself. I'm around beautiful women all the time, but it doesn't matter because Christy has learned to capture my mind. The other day I was traveling and found a card in my suitcase. Cool. We all love surprises. Let me read you the front of the card. "Sometimes when I look at you, I wonder how I got so lucky." Ladies swoon at this kind of stuff. You know how guys feel about it? It means nothing to a guy. But here's the part where she captured my mind: when I opened that card, right in the middle was a piece of her lingerie. All day long, I was thinking about her. That entire trip all I was thinking about was her. She's not stupid. She knows how this works. She left that little piece of fabric there for me and captured my mind. It doesn't matter who I meet or what comes up throughout the rest of my day, she has all of my mind. I can't wait to see her again. Why? She's leveraging my testosterone and helping me stay a healthy man. Ladies you can cause a man to be deeply focused on you and chase you the rest of your life if you just do those four things. Here's the best part—you also keep him healthy. It may sound tough or like something you may not want to do, but how much do each of these first four steps cost? Trust me, the care from our clinics is much more expensive. You don't want to have to pay us to help you get your man's testosterone back to normal. These steps cost you nothing, just a little understanding and creativity.

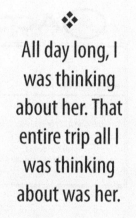

All day long, I was thinking about her. That entire trip all I was thinking about was her.

#5 TEST THE BOY

I often get emails and phone calls from women who have tried #1-4 to tell me it didn't work. Well, then #5 is very important. You need to make sure you get tested. I had a thirty-one-year-old man and his wife come into my office. Over the course of the last three years he had lost his job, gained a lot of weight and had zero motivation. Most notably, no sexual drive. It had been two years since he'd had sex with his wife. Does that sound like a healthy boy? His wife looked at me and said, "If I wasn't a Christian woman, I would have left him already.

All I have is a roommate. I don't want a roommate. I want a husband."
I asked him if he had ever had his hormones tested. You can guess
what his answer was. No. But do you know what they did have him
on? SIX anti-depressants. In our current way of thinking, the thought
was he might have a tumor or fire of some kind. They found nothing,
and since they weren't going to cut him open, it was time to use the
hose. They kept adding medications. He was finally on six prescribed
medications and in a horrible state! I did the obvious and measured
his hormones. I sent him to the hospital where he was getting his
psychiatric treatments. Take a look at his levels here:

Access
MEDICAL LABS

5151 CORPORATE WAY
JUPITER, FL 33458-3101
(866)720-8386

Client: THE WELLNESS WAY 11118	Patient:		
2638 TULIP LN	Room#	DOB. ( ) -	Age: Sex: M
SUITE B	Phone:		
GREEN BAY, WI 54313	ID#:		
Phys: FLYNN, PATRICK	Route#:		Page: 1

ENDOCRINE EVALUATION			
DHEA-SULFATE	68.5	34.5 – 568.9	ug/dl
DIHYDROTESTOSTERONE	12.2	11.2 – 95.5	ng/dL
TESTOSTERONE, TOTAL	0.0 L	280 – 1100	ng/dl
SEX HORMONE BIND GLOBULIN	16 L	21.63 – 113.1	nmol/L
Lab Developed Testing	********		

Can you see his levels? No? Because they are 0! Zero. I called the
hospital to see if they had made a mistake. They had him come back in
and checked it four times. Four. It was consistently the same. Zero. We
figured out what triggered his fires and what he needed to rebuild his
house. After three months, we ran his blood work:

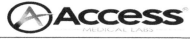

Client: THE WELLNESS WAY		11118	Patient:		
2638 TULIP LN			Room#	DOB.	Age: Sex:M
SUITE B			Phone:		Fasting:
GREEN BAY, WI 54313			ID#:		
Phys: FLYNN, PATRICK			Route#: 0		Page:1

ENDOCRINE EVALUATION				
TESTOSTERONE, TOTAL	717	280 – 1100	ng/dl
SEX HORMONE BIND GLOBULIN	39	10 – 80	nmol/L
TESTOSTERONE, FREE	13.98	1.9 – 27	ng/dl

I had them come in to go over his labs. This time his wife's first words to me were, "Doc, turn it off!" His body had gone back to normal. We like to see numbers anywhere over 400 Ng/dL for men's testosterone levels to be in the Man Zone. Ladies, I have received flack for this next statement, but like I said, I speak it like it is. If your husband is not chasing you every day, it's a sign he's sick. I don't care if he's sixty or if he's twenty-five. If he's chasing you every day, he's not a pervert. He's a real healthy man and you should be thanking God for that. Guys are easy to understand, easy to get back to normal and easy to keep normal. We have a simple daily and lifelong cycle.

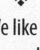

We like to see numbers anywhere over 400 Ng/dL for men's testosterone levels to be in the Man Zone.

CHRISTY'S THOUGHTS

If only women realized that the four steps really worked and were so incredibly beneficial to men's health!! I didn't even realize that I was doing those four steps until he started pointing them out to me, or until he started using examples in his seminars. You can imagine the look on my face after I heard him bring up the 'lingerie in the card' in one of his seminars for the first time—I was probably redder than a lobster, and I guarantee my eyes were as wide as saucers!! But ladies, in all seriousness, I can handle a small bit of embarrassment if I know that it will help you with your marriage! The best advice I have for ladies to build and keep their men and marriages healthy is to do these four steps! Ladies, we need to help our men stay hormone-healthy 'till death do us part'.

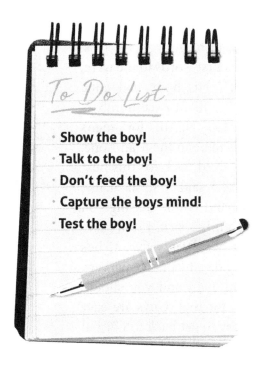

To Do List

- **Show the boy!**
- **Talk to the boy!**
- **Don't feed the boy!**
- **Capture the boys mind!**
- **Test the boy!**

CHAPTER 8

GRRR

I wake up early in the morning to get to work on my priorities; I usually make it to the office before everyone else. I make myself a cup of good, organic coffee and sit down to read e-mails back in the studio. One day, I opened a message from a man who was frustrated. His wife was exhausted, she can't get out of bed any more, and she has been bleeding for over two months. The doctors couldn't find anything wrong with her.

What I read every morning frustrates me. It actually makes me sad. I sit down every morning to e-mails from women from all over the world who are sick. They are sick and aren't getting any help from the doctors charged with their care. They have been told to accept what they are experiencing as normal. This is personal for me because my wife was once one of those women. So, early in the morning reading all these e-mails, that's when I might get upset and go on a rant to tell people there's a different perspective! There's a different way of thinking traditional medicine doesn't have! Can you blame me? Women's illness and hormone problems have skyrocketed through the years.

Doctors are not trying to *not* help. They are trying to do the best job they can. That doesn't take away the fact that women are sick, and they are in pain. However, their job is to keep them alive, not help them live their best life with an optimally functioning body. The current method is so incomplete that my heart breaks when they come in. Women have been to so many doctors by the time they come in to see us. We are usually the last resort because we aren't part of the huge medical machine. I ask for their records and the most basic things when they come in. It is always incomplete testing that doesn't give a good picture of what is happening with them. It doesn't matter if they've been to an M.D., D.O., endocrinologist, functional medicine doctor or other specialists. Their testing is incomplete, because they simply were not taught complete testing. To assess a woman properly is impossible if you are trying to do it with a limited perspective.

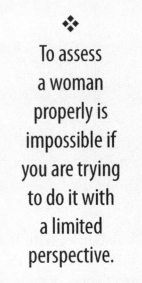

❖
To assess a woman properly is impossible if you are trying to do it with a limited perspective.

Have you been at the movies watching the previews when you saw a preview to a movie that looked really good? Then you think *we have to see that*. You make a date to see the movie. A few months later, you go to the movie and it's meh. You judged the movie on the preview and you only got a small picture of what that movie was about. We have all been to a movie that had a pretty good preview, but it was bad when you saw the whole thing. We understand the preview is just a small picture. Unfortunately, that's how traditional medicine is looking at women's hormones.

You were never taught how a woman's hormones work and we wonder why breast cancer rates are rising. We wonder why there are so many hormonal issues. If you are like most Americans, you most likely haven't been educated on how a woman's body works. That's ok, we're fixing that right now. How many of you have heard of the hormone estrogen? You ready for this? There is no such thing as the hormone estrogen. Estrogen is a term for ten different hormones that are chemically similar. They may be chemically similar, but they have different properties. With how much high estrogen is connected to increased risk of breast cancer, it seems we should get to the bottom of this. Pink ribbons, mammograms and all the research for drugs can't give you *prevention*. Understanding the multiple hormones and proper testing can set your body up for health. This group of hormones control if you get cancer, osteoporosis, and/or heart disease. Estrogens even control your moods—whether you are happy or depressed. Like I said, they play an important part of making up who a woman is!

Women who have been diagnosed with breast cancer will be tested to see if their type of cancer is estrogen <u>positive</u>. If the results say their cancer type is estrogen <u>receptive</u>, they will be put on an aromatase inhibiting drug that blocks their production of all estrogens. It's non-selective so that means it stops the production and conversion of <u>all</u> the estrogens. Not just the problematic one. If you understand that each estrogen has a unique role, then you understand how damaging this can be. One of those estrogens, 2-hydroxy Estrone, is actually cancer *protective*. That's just one of them and you have ten!

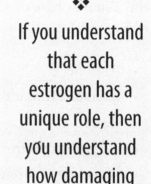

If you understand that each estrogen has a unique role, then you understand how damaging this can be.

All of the estrogens play an important role in your body and making a woman who she is. Estrogen is demonized just because one type of estrogen gets out of control which can create an environment that allows breast cancer to grow and spread. Demonizing estrogen can have a detrimental effect on a body that relies on multiple estrogens for health.

The other problem is, you should be thinking about how estrogen impacts your health before you have breast cancer. Why aren't we doing more to make sure women are set up for their best hormonal health? A mammogram won't prevent breast cancer. It helps identify breast cancer but doesn't stop it! You need to get all of your estrogen hormones tested properly. That starts by knowing there is more than one.

Have you had all of those hormones tested? I ask this question all over the country when I speak and in my practice. Unless they are going to a Wellness Way Clinic, they have not had their hormones tested properly.

You may have had one or two hormones tested, but have you had all of them? You may have thought you have; but unless you have been to a Wellness Way you probably haven't. Here's what you need to get tested:

- Estrone
- Estradiol (this is the major one tested for)
- Estriol
- 16-hydroxy Estrone
- 4-hydroxy Estrone
- 2-hydroxy Estrone
- 2-methoxy Estrone

I have an idea. If the only thing that triggers the breast cancer gene is out of control estrogens, why don't we check all of the estrogen levels when women are at a young age. That makes sense.

Estrogens dictate your life, not just your breast cancer risk. It's better to prevent illness than to treat illness. I don't treat breast cancer. I am not equipped to do so. If you have breast cancer, you should go to the fire department doctor. But I have a question, why would we treat breast cancer if we could *protect* you from getting breast cancer by supporting hormonal health?

My wife had horrible health problems and painful periods. The medical community told her she would most likely not have been able to bear children. She saw lots of doctors. When I tested these hormones in my wife, I found out one of them turned her uterus into pathological disease. When we got that hormone normal, her uterus went back to normal. We lowered her risk for breast cancer by supporting her hormones, her health problems subsided, and her periods became normal. Testing your hormones can change your health and your life. Do you think her doctors tested her hormones completely? No.

If your doctor has just tested your blood, there is no way you can get a true picture of all your hormones. There are three ways to test your hormones. To get a full understanding of your hormonal health you need to utilize more than one test.

- Blood
- Saliva
- Urine

Let me say this again so you can share with your gynecologist, your nurse practitioner, your doctor and anyone else who just wants to draw your blood to test your hormones: it is virtually impossible to get a full picture of your hormonal health by testing blood alone. The main hormone they can look at through blood testing is estradiol. Conveniently, this is one they can manipulate through drugs. If you

It is virtually impossible to get a full picture of your hormonal health by testing blood alone.

haven't had a urine test to check your hormones, you are missing important indicators. There are certain estrogens you can only see in urine. But you can't test progesterone in a urine test, so for a full hormonal picture you will need multiple tests. I can't say this enough; a good clinical doctor will run multiple tests to get a full picture. Now think about it—did you know about the ten estrogens? Did you get multiple types of testing?

CHRISTY'S THOUGHTS

> Yes, I did all three hormone tests within the same timeframe to get the proper "picture" of what was going on in my body. Everyone is different, and I cannot stress enough how important it is to get all your hormones tested and get the 'whole picture'! I have done it multiple times through the years, and my daughters will also get testing done as soon as they each begin menstruating. There is no going back to the 'common' way of doing things for us...remember, I went to other doctors and did all their testing and got NO results and NO answers. As a result of testing thoroughly through The Wellness Way, both my life and my daughters' lives have been put on a path leading to homeostasis and away from disease. Testing is key!

Using the standard approach, women are left with incomplete information and trusting people who are looking at an incomplete picture of the body. And we wonder why hormone conditions, hormonal problems, and breast cancer continue to rise. We have a hormone problem in this country that leads to high breast cancer rates. People are racing for the cure, buying the pink ribbon version of everything, attending rallies, and participating in pink 5k races–we know we have a problem, and people clearly want to help. However, imagine if this information I just shared with you was brought into the conversation. We are missing the discussions that can really lead to saving lives and improved quality of health. When you understand how estrogens work and how to properly test, we can do more for prevention. It's part of a whole-body approach that understands whether you are setting your body up for health or illness.

When you start supporting a body for healthy hormones and healthy systems, your body starts responding with positive outcomes. There is more to it than just learning the names of the hormones though. Not only do women have more hormones, these hormones are changing on a regular basis. Let's take a look at a chart of the typical woman's cycle.

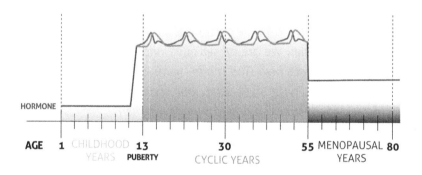

Looks quite a bit different from the graphic we looked at on men's hormones, huh?

Would you agree with me that testosterone alone causes physical and mental changes? Women have a lot more hormones that change throughout the month, not just throughout the day. Their cycles are very different. Their cycle and hormones affect them differently than men, both physically and mentally. Looking at the charts of the hormones, can you understand how I question how can anybody tell us that men and women are the same? I believe the lack of understanding of hormones is causing many of our common problems today. Even during counseling, a man is often told to be more sensitive. If a man is healthy and his testosterone levels are good, this is going to be very hard for him to do. It's denying his biology! Men are not supposed to be overly sensitive. That's not what they are. Conversely, women are supposed to be sensitive, and their hormones make their experience different than a man's. Their emotions do not mean they are crazy, it's their biology!

Understanding the different hormones and how they work can not only support a woman's health, it can improve her relationships.

CHRISTY'S THOUGHTS

One of the most beneficial pieces of advice I ever got was to not discuss difficult things or topics with Patrick during the day, but instead to wait…to 'bridle my tongue' and talk to him at night about the issue. Ladies, we are all sensitive and emotional, but they are NOT—and that's how God made them! It's not wrong, so why not THINK DIFFERENTLY and change our approach to solving problems, instead of constantly trying to change our men??

Approach your man in the evening when his testosterone is lower and remember that it's not what you say, but HOW you say it. Speak respectfully, and he will be more likely to respond back respectfully. Your tone of voice can actually say more than you are trying to say. You could be completely right, but how you say something can determine whether he receives it or not. So, don't try to make him more 'sensitive'! He's a man, and a healthy man has testosterone. If we could all (men and women) learn to control our reactions, I think conflict resolution would not be so dreaded or difficult.

Amanda's Story

I had been pretty healthy in my teen years. I had no challenges with my cycles. Everything seemed just fine. The challenges started after I decided to go off my birth control—Depo-Provera injections.

I struggled with stage IV endometriosis and cysts for about 10 years. I felt like I lived a double life. With endometriosis I looked like every other happy and healthy person on the outside. However, at home I spent most of my time with a heating pad and on high doses of pain medication. I hated to tell anyone how I was feeling. I often felt like I was viewed as broken or just making up the symptoms. Endometriosis is a very lonely disease. It drained me both physically and mentally. I felt like a burden causing my family to miss out on so many opportunities. My husband was very supportive and stayed by my side through it all.

I tried every medication to the maximum limits – even to the point of signing waiver forms for these higher doses – had my uterus scraped yearly and was in a hopeless situation. During one emergency surgery, the doctor thought the challenge was my appendix and removed it. My appendix was actually fine. I felt like an experiment to the doctors I was seeing.

Everything we tried seemed to work for a month or so before the pain returned full force. The doctors had no more answers or treatments to try. We were out of options, except for a drastic hysterectomy, and even then, I couldn't be guaranteed a pain free life. All the courses of action we had taken had damaged my body more than helped. I am still challenged with some of the side effects of the drugs I had been given.

I found myself at my chiropractor's office, desperate for help. I was ready to try anything. When my chiropractor reached out to

Dr. Patrick to consult, he looked at my tests and asked if I was a 60-year-old woman in menopause. I was a 31-year-old woman. After starting my Wellness Way journey, I was pain free after 3 months! My chiropractor was so impacted, he became a Wellness Way affiliate, so he would be able to help others.

I haven't had any medication or surgery in over two years and I'm not looking back now. In fact, I would be afraid to go back to my previous doctor—the one who "accidentally" took out my appendix. I'm afraid I would be kicked out for how strongly I feel about my health and the hope The Wellness Way has restored in my life.

It wasn't always easy, but you must to do the right thing for your health. I have a supportive husband, but still had a lot of criticism from those who didn't understand what I was doing and choosing. I had to choose to stay the course and do the right thing for my family, for my health.

I share my story hoping that it helps others find the help they need. I don't want anyone to have to go through the life of pain and misery, so many health challenges can cause, especially in the way of female hormones. I feel better at 33 then I did in my 20's. Thanks to The Wellness Way Approach I have my life back, and I know they can do that for so many more people!

Chapter 9

Women Are Complicated, but Worth It

This chapter is a bit longer than the one on the man zone. Women have more hormones and more zones. They are a bit more complicated than a man; that is what makes them women.

When I started researching women's hormones, one question kept jumping out at me and caused me to focus all my research on answering it. Why do women care about everything? Why do they look at everything the way they do? Let's take a day in the life of a woman. From the time a woman gets up in the morning, she is the primary person to get the kids ready for school. Have you ever seen a guy dress his kids? My wife always asks me, "how could you possibly let them leave the house dressed like that?" Sure, they might look funny but I think: it's fine, they have clothes on. Done! We think differently. Moms make breakfast, pack lunches, ready the kids for school and then drop them off. Then moms pour themselves into a multitude of tasks all day, at home, the office, or both. Then after school they take care of

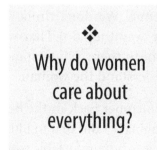

❖

Why do women care about everything?

the kids and have to make food again, help with homework and after they've cared for everything all day long, they are exhausted. But this intense schedule means so much to her because it's what she does. She cares. About everything!

Now, her man left this morning and he cared about what? Nothing! Ok, that's not to mean he doesn't care about *anything*, but remember, his testosterone keeps him laser-focused on one thing. He's got his "one thing" on his mind and is moving through the day. One thing at a time, one task conquered after another. He's doing great, he thinks! Triumphant, he heads home at the end of his day. What is that guy thinking when he comes home? (Insert sexy music here.)

And how does the woman respond? "Just another thing I have to do!" It's comical looking at the two perspectives, isn't it? Ladies, I hear you. This is the story you've told me for eighteen years. Guys—just understand, it's a thing. It happens and it's real. They are different from us. It's okay to be a man, but you have to understand women are very different; and it's okay to be a woman. Their hormones make them more emotional. They think differently; they care about everything. We don't. Our testosterone keeps us less emotional and only thinking about one thing at a time. We don't think about ten things the way they do. That whole day means a lot to them. Understand that and you'll understand the woman.

> ❖
> **It's okay to be a man, but you have to understand women are very different; and it's okay to be a woman.**

Remember back in the beginning of the book when I used the word "vagina?" I did that to illustrate a point. To understand each other, we have to be comfortable with some basics, but it's going to be tricky when the basics make many men squeamish. Women, have you ever noticed a large population of men are interested in hunting? In Wisconsin, we live in a hunting state, so men and women get this analogy. A guy can go to Cabela's, buy deer urine and spray it all over himself and the trees. He can go fishing and scrape the scales off the fish and clean them without batting an eye. He can kill a deer with either a gun or bow and field dress it right there in the woods with very few tools. But the minute a woman says she has her cycle, he's grossed out. Ever notice that? The irony is funny! Now this isn't every man, but I do come across it often. Guys, I know I caught your attention with the "v word", but I won't make you uncomfortable. I promise I won't use the word vagina anymore. Don't worry, we'll still communicate effectively.

Let's go back to my analogy, and use the example of a house. For the rest of the section, we'll look at the female cycle through a man's point of view. If a female is a house in this analogy, we'll call the word I promised not to say "the Man Cave." Not because the man owns it! Rather, of all the places in the house a man may enjoy, the Man Cave is his favorite spot. Men love going to their Man Caves—it makes them happy. In this house, the Man Cave changes on a regular basis. Why? There are physical and mental changes going on. All the time. This is what a cycle looks like for a woman through the course of a month:

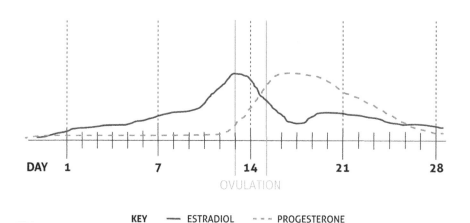

DAY 1 7 14 21 28

OVULATION

KEY — ESTRADIOL - - - PROGESTERONE

A woman's cycle can range from twenty-six to thirty-two days and it's okay. It can be twenty-seven one time and twenty-nine another. It doesn't have to be the exact same every time. The average cycle for women is about twenty-eight days. Let's look at the hormone patterns. These patterns change on a woman four times a month. When I got married, my wife looked at me after our pastor said our vows and said, "I do." Guys, it's different for us. The pastor should have asked us to say, "I do" four times. When you say, "I do" to a woman, you are really marrying four different women. I'm going to show you how this works and it's not as weird as it may sound. Have you ever noticed sometimes your wife can be really awesome and then the following week all you are thinking is *who did I marry?!* You think she's a totally different person. Guys, you know it's true, but you also have to know that sometimes, the personality shift is just fine and even okay. Men (and women) don't understand so they think there's something wrong with them when this happens. And when the man tells her she has to be like him, it only makes it worse. Today's sexual revolution is telling us that women can be as sexually driven as men. Please don't—they can't and they shouldn't. If they are as driven as men, they are sick. Let me say it again. If a woman has a sex drive like a man, she is sick and will probably develop cancer someday. Let me explain the woman zones.

Zone 1: The Construction Zone

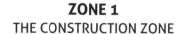

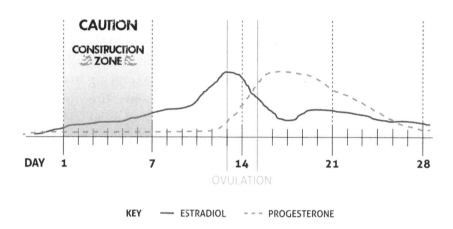

ZONE 1
THE CONSTRUCTION ZONE

KEY ⎯ ESTRADIOL - - - PROGESTERONE

This is when the cycle starts. The cycle can go anywhere from four to seven days. This is when the Man Cave is under construction. Her hormones change, and the first two weeks of her cycle are dominated by estrogens.

Estrogens make a woman who she is, just like testosterone makes guys who we are. But let's come back to one thing—if this is what makes each of us who we are, estrogens for women, and testosterone for men—how many of us have had them tested? They make up so much of who we are. The method of the fire department is to not worry about anything until your house is on fire. I want to see normal hormones and keep it that way and therefore preventing fires. The only way to know if they are normal is to have them

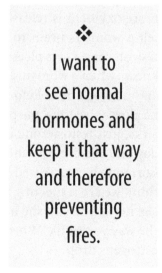

❖

I want to see normal hormones and keep it that way and therefore preventing fires.

tested and then to take care of them throughout their cycle. So, the construction zone is a very important time during a woman's cycle and keeping hormones healthy. The body is under a certain amount of stress because it is in construction. It takes work and resources for the body to properly undergo this process.

When we test, we are working to keep tabs on those levels and prevent, or help our patients recover from the devastation of disease, or fire that could result. When someone's body is trying to adapt to stress their body could have trouble making or converting hormones. Simply stated, those hormones are getting thrown off. However, until you develop cancer, and your house is actually on fire, the fire department won't show up. By the time cancer is detected, it's been growing for years!

Estrogens are produced by the ovaries. That's important, because later in the month this hormone production will change. What do estrogens do for women? They make them energetic, outgoing, social, enthusiastic, alters their metabolism, and they eat about 15% less than men. It also increases their serotonin—the happy hormone.

Men, pay attention. When the Man Cave is under construction, more oxytocin is released, and her love hormone goes up. Estrogens tell a woman's brain to connect. They don't say "go get it" like your testosterone. Guys please learn this—it will be life-changing. Every guy knows when a woman starts her cycle and the Man Cave is unavailable and he won't be able to visit it anytime soon. He disconnects because he doesn't see the purpose. Again ladies, this is not because we are jerks, just testosterone driven, focus-on-the-moment guys. But guys, day one of a cycle is where you can make your wife very sick. Her love hormone has increased and because our sex drive can't be fulfilled, we think we are respecting her by not "pestering." Fair thought. However, she needs you and she needs you in a very specific way, maybe just not the way you think. When you separate from her, her love hormone and estrogens drop.

We have to understand, guys, it's okay for you to have a sex drive, but this is how her body works so you have to put her needs above yours during this zone. Your sex drive will still be there when it's over, and you want her to be healthy. When her cycle comes, it's your job to work at connecting with her. This is key to keeping her healthy. Ask her how her day was and what's happening in her life. If she just says everything is fine, then dig a little deeper. Do things that she enjoys doing. I take my wife dancing, but that might not be what your wife likes. Do what she likes. Watch the romantic comedy, take a walk with her, fix her favorite dinner, or whatever it is she likes. The most important thing is that she feels connected to you and knows that you understand her.

Here's an interesting tidbit about working out. Ladies, if you exercise during The Construction Zone, you run the risk of draining your hormones and pushing your body to be stressed. Your body then thinks it has to produce more hormone. There is one tissue that does a really good job of making hormone—fat. Yes, the very thing you are trying to avoid! Brutal! Another reason why understanding your physiology is important. If you push your body during the wrong times of the month during the wrong zones you can exercise all you want, and you'll gain more fat.

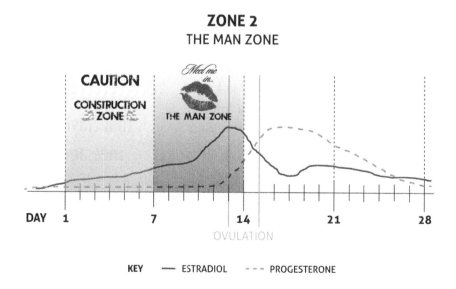

ZONE 2
THE MAN ZONE

CAUTION

CONSTRUCTION ZONE

Meet me in...

THE MAN ZONE

DAY 1   7   14   21   28

OVULATION

KEY   — ESTRADIOL   - - - PROGESTERONE

Zone 2: The Man Zone

When the cycle stops, and her hormones have come up properly, she enters the zone eager men are waiting for. She becomes just like a man in her sex drive. A woman in her Zone 1 doesn't have much of a sex drive, but as everything increases, so does that libido. It's okay and very normal for her sex drive to match her man's at this time. Let's look at those estrogens and how to support them again. This is the week to exercise. In the Man Zone, it's very important for ladies to exercise. Their bodies can handle it. They also handle stress better, it may even seem like nothing bothers them. Women also burn sugar better in this zone. Have you noticed there are times when you can eat anything and not gain a pound and other times you eat an organic salad and gain five? It's probably the same week your husband gives up soda and loses twenty pounds. We know—it's annoying.

Men, this is the week to help feed her body the right way. We're talking about serotonin, fatty acid, estrogen-based foods. Let's picture a stressed-out woman. Her day was terrible, her husband was frustrating, work was horrible, her kids are driving her nuts and she's craving an organic salad. Does that sound right to you? No! I've never heard a woman say that. When you are stressed, what does your body crave? Chocolate! Do you know why? Chocolate has the highest serotonin content of any food on the planet. Your body knew exactly what it was doing when it sent that craving message.

Your body knew exactly what it was doing when it sent that craving message.

When I started understanding this, I studied chocolate like crazy. Hershey still sells more chocolate than anyone else in the world. Valentine's Day, February 14, four *billion* Hershey's kisses are sold! When I'm talking about the health benefits of chocolate, I'm not talking about Hershey or any other highly-processed chocolate–those are filled with sugar and chemicals. I'm talking about healthy, real food. Raw cacao is actually a superfood with a ton of benefits. There's a very big difference between it and what you can find on display by the register at the grocery store. Don't reach for the bad stuff. That isn't the message your body is sending!

Men, here's a valuable "insider secret", if you will. There are many different forms of chocolate. There are cacao beans, nibs, powder, paste, but let me tell you about a little gem called cacao *butter*. You should feel my hands. They're pretty nice for a guy's hands. Let me tell you why. I'll take some cacao butter and coconut oil and when my wife gets her cycle, I'll start rubbing her down and massaging her. Why? Because I'm a nice guy? Well, I'm nice, but giving massages isn't exactly my favorite pastime. But I understand how cacao benefits my wife, so I'm trying to make sure that while she's under the Construction Zone, I'm going to do everything I can to get her into the Man Zone and keep her in the Man Zone. I rub her down and feed her body by rubbing healthy oils and fats on her skin. My hands are so nice because I understand it's my role as her husband to help her through Zone 1 so we can get to Zone 2 and make sure Zone 2 is as good as it can be. Guys, we do have it easy. We keep our testosterone good and things are really simple for us. It's very difficult for a woman. Their bodies change four times in a month. FOUR! I keep saying it, and I will until every man and woman realizes this is normal, not crazy.

> ❖
> It's very difficult for a woman. Their bodies change four times in a month.

Think differently. By looking at things from a different perspective, we can help you figure out what specifically each woman needs. We want husbands to understand this as well because as your body is going through that transition, he should help you with this. You are a team, and, up until now, I suspect that no one has ever taught you how to support each other's hormone health.

Women turn to me when their hormones show their bodies are in distress. That's how I end up with a baseball-sized blood clot on my desk? Ok, I'm a doctor and all, and totally comfortable with anatomy but this was a doozy even for me! A patient I was working with who had endometriosis came into my office just after her period started and placed a plastic baggie with a giant blood clot in it on my desk.

Yes, a plastic baggie.

Yes, a baseball-sized blood clot. I can still picture it.

She asked me, "What do you think about that?"

I paused, then slowly said, "Well…I don't think it belongs on my desk…!"

We laughed but despite the humor, her situation wasn't funny. You see, I didn't need to see the enormous clot to understand the pain she was experiencing. I have supported, and continue to support, many women who are facing similar experiences. She knew I dealt with these types of issues all the time, so she trusted me enough to bring in her clot. I responded by helping her get her hormones back in shape and guiding her back to homeostasis.

There is a lot you can learn when women trust you and share their experiences with you.

I had a woman come in who was dealing with what I'll call "Man Cave Dryness," (you know what I mean). She sent me an email after I figured out what her body needed, and she started taking steps to correct her situation. Here's the email:

> Dr. Patrick, I wanted to update you and thank you for the advice you gave my husband and me at our last appointment. When you told me the benefits of coconut oil and cacao butter, and how it affects the vaginal tissue, I thought you were a little bit crazy. But you've given me good advice so far, so we decided to try it. After applying it vaginally for a couple of days, we started to notice that the soreness started to go down, so we decided to try it out. After a couple of weeks, I'm happy to tell you that I'm starting to enjoy sex again and my husband is very pleased. Not just because we've had more sex in the last couple of weeks than we've had in the last year, but my husband and I have been able to get into positions that I have not been in for over thirty years. He thanks you! Your advice has helped me physically, mentally and brought me closer to my husband.

She's eighty-three years young. Can you believe it? It goes to show your body is meant to function optimally no matter what your age is.

Alright guys, here's the first of your two To Do Lists:

#1 FEED THE GIRL

I'm going to help you guys read a woman's mind. Not all of it; testosterone or no, we aren't equipped for that! Here is the most important thing that you can help with on a regular basis, "Feed me chocolate and tell me I'm pretty." She needs the chocolate and loves the reassurance. Remember she doesn't have testosterone telling her how

❖

Remember she doesn't have testosterone telling her how awesome she is.

awesome she is. It's your job to tell her. It was part of the marriage agreement when you said, "I do" to your four wives.

Ladies, if you fast, you'll be very sick. Feed the hormones. For a guy you need to starve their hormones; this is just one more way we are very different. That's why women can eat hardly anything and still be overweight. Men, in the first two weeks of their cycle, help them with this. Provide the things they need to feed their hormones. They need it—the results will prove it to you. People are blown away because after doing the most simple and basic things, their bodies begin changing like crazy. During the first two weeks of her cycle, a woman needs to be eating foods high in fatty acids. Here's your shopping list:

- Chocolate-the good kind!
- Chia seeds
- Pumpkin seeds
- Sunflower seeds
- Coconut products
- Walnuts
- Pecans and most other nuts
- Olive oil
- Hemp
- Dates
- Avocados
- Cherries
- Grapes (organic wine is okay)
- Maca

Some essential oils that may also help during this time are thyme, lemon and patchouli.

#2 TALK TO THE GIRL

Now that the ladies have read the first part of the book, the guys are loving life. Their ladies are taking care of them and understand how their guys work. If guys are confused, they may walk up to their ladies in the morning (because they think their lady is just like them) and say "honey, tonight is going to be a good night!" Guess what is going to happen. Your wife is NOT going to come home that night. Why? That doesn't connect with a woman. Don't speak to a woman that way—they need more finesse! We see the idea of "guy phrases" in movies and while guys think

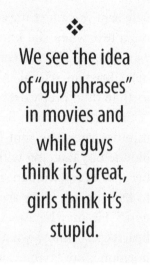

We see the idea of "guy phrases" in movies and while guys think it's great, girls think it's stupid.

it's great, girls think it's stupid. They know that's not how it works. That doesn't appeal to a woman. Women need connecting words.

There are three words that appeal to a woman. Guys may think it doesn't matter, because she knows it already, but ask my wife. I tell her this all the time. I text her this phrase early in the morning and I'll text it to her in the afternoon. What are the three most important words you can say to a woman?

Hint: it's not "I love you."

It's "I choose you." That is one of the most connecting things you can say to a woman. When you disconnect from her, she feels left alone. When she feels disconnected, she'll create things in her head. When you disconnect with her, she thinks you're connecting with someone else. She really does. And she'll play it over in her head and she'll create scenarios and the weirdest things you will ever hear in your life. Most of us have been through it.

About six months ago as I was getting ready to speak to a group, my wife sent me a text message. I thought that was odd, she doesn't send me a text when she knows I'm getting ready to go on stage. But this was special. My thirteen-year-old daughter was at her first dance at her Christian school. All the girls were standing, swaying back and forth in their pretty dresses. What do you think they were all thinking? "Come, choose me!" To women this is sweet and precious. Then, two minutes later, she sent me a picture with this cute thirteen-year-old blonde boy dancing with my daughter. It meant so much to my wife, because every woman, my wife included, knows how important it is to feel chosen. Guys are different so all I could think is, "where's my gun?" He may be sweet, but I turned into protective Papa Bear in a heartbeat! I know what those pubescent boys are like and what his hormones are saying... anyway! Back to the ladies. Every woman loves to be pursued, to know that she is the focus of her man's affection. It's in their biology. Guys, when you don't chase them, they start to feel disconnected from you.

I've made an observation. Watch out for your friends, ladies. When one of them goes through a divorce or another stressful time, no matter the age, they get very sick quickly. They just do. When a woman feels disconnected and goes through a bad relationship, her hormones drop. Ladies, here's a tip. When your friend is going through a lot of stress, sometimes women can pick up the slack where men are not. That's sad, isn't it? Your friends can help you out just by being a connecting friend. Guys, you can't help each other out that way. Our testosterone won't be driven up by connecting to another man. We're not wired that way.

CHRISTY'S THOUGHTS

To be chosen…over and over again…it's the most amazing feeling, isn't it? You know what we do every day to keep our relationship playful and alive? Patrick and I have our own 'code' that we send each other via emojis! Between emojis and GIFs, we stay connected all throughout each day, even when we are so busy, we don't have time to talk. Be creative and playful in your relationships and you will be pleasantly surprised by how close you become. And ladies, you can be an ear to listen to your girlfriends when they are going through stress. Just listen and connect, and you will help reduce her stress.

One piece of advice from what I have observed though…ladies, if you are struggling in your marriage, guard your heart and do not talk and connect with other men. Ladies should connect with ladies, and guys should talk to guys when it comes to marriage issues and counseling. Just as my husband mentioned in the chapter on testosterone…guys, if you stress your woman out and you don't go out of your way to try to connect with her and she starts talking and connecting with another man, you may be heading in a dangerous direction of destruction in your marriage. Three little words: I Choose You…or Connect, Connect, Connect, can mean the difference between a healthy vibrant marriage and one that is stagnant and dysfunctional. Love is a verb…you need to choose to actively love your spouse in the way that they receive it best!

#3 Touch the Girl

I have gotten thousands of emails on this one.

Guys, the light switches for the Man Cave are not inside the Man Cave. Simple as that.

A woman changes four times a month. Finding the light switches can be an adventure. They move every week. It's like looking for Waldo in a different place

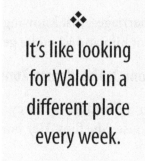

❖

It's like looking for Waldo in a different place every week.

every week. You know this, because you think, *I've got this. It was a good night. I touched her there and she loved it.* Next week you go to touch her there and she's all: "DON'T touch me!" She's not crazy. Her body changed. One area that was sensitive and felt good one week doesn't feel as good the following week. Guys, when they touch us, it feels good all the time. Right? Just make it a game and try to find those light switches. I've had emails that have said it's changed people's

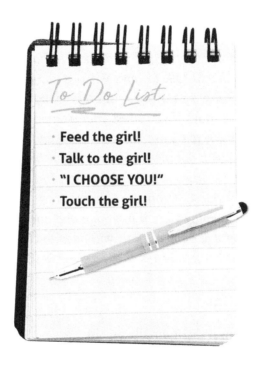

marriages, just knowing they each like to be touched differently. She's not him and when he gets that, they're both good.

Zone 3: The Woman Zone

In the middle of her cycle, you have a totally different woman in your house. She flips. Her hormones are totally different.

Ladies, hear this clearly: you are normal. You ladies will come to me because your emotions change, and you feel bad. Please—you don't need to feel bad! Just like your husband has no control over his morning testosterone, you have no control over your hormones and emotions changing. None. That should give you ladies a lot of mental

ZONE 3
THE WOMAN ZONE

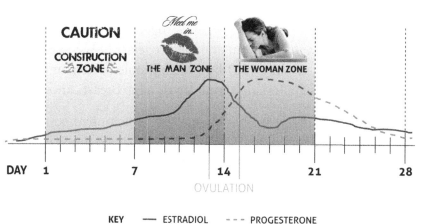

KEY   —— ESTRADIOL   - - - PROGESTERONE

peace. You are not supposed to have your emotions flat lined. It's okay for you to go up and down. There's nothing wrong with that. Look what happens in Zone 3:

Be very careful guys, you don't know who you are coming home to during this zone. I mean this sincerely, she may bite you. Ok, not literally! Just know she's normal. Don't make her feel bad because she's emotional and her body is more sensitive to these changes.

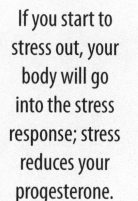

❖

If you start to stress out, your body will go into the stress response; stress reduces your progesterone.

With the switch of the hormones, her adrenals take over instead of the ovaries we talked about the first half of the cycle. These are the stress glands. If your body hasn't been adjusted, has chemical stress, and physical stress and you are emotionally stressed out, this is the week that will make you very sick. If you exercise too hard during this week, it will make you sick. Your body needs to relax. If you start to stress out, your body will go into the stress response; stress reduces your progesterone. Have you heard of the hormone progesterone? Yes, it's just one hormone. I'm not trying to trick you here. The main job of progesterone is to balance what estrogens do. Progesterone is a calming hormone, and stress can drain it. Progesterone takes estrogens and balances them so they don't become a problem. Remember how we said if estrogens get too high, you can develop breast cancer?

Let's look at a seventy-year-old patient. This woman had gone to her medical doctor and by the time she had gotten to us she was only taking two anti-depressants. She wanted to get off them because she felt she was getting worse. Her son, who is in his fifties, brought her into our office. We had changed his life and he knew we could help her. She had gone through all the tests and exams her general practitioner would

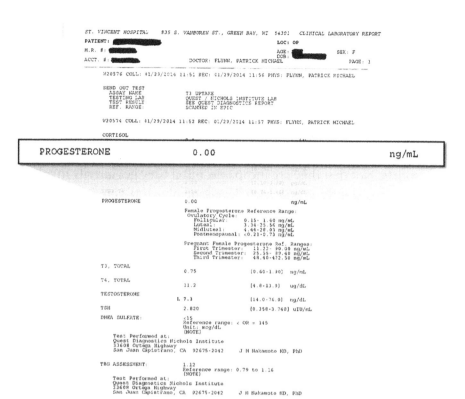

```
ST. VINCENT HOSPITAL    835 S. VANBUREN ST., GREEN BAY, WI  54301   CLINICAL LABORATORY REPORT
   PATIENT:                                  LOC: OP
   M.R. #:                                   AGE:            SEX: F
   ACCT. #:                DOCTOR: FLYNN, PATRICK MICHAEL    DOB:        PAGE: 1

      W20576 COLL: 01/29/2014 11:51 REC: 01/29/2014 11:56 PHYS: FLYNN, PATRICK MICHAEL

      SEND OUT TEST
       ASSAY NAME      T3 UPTAKE
       TESTING LAB     QUEST / NICHOLS INSTITUTE LAB
       TEST RESULT     SEE QUEST DIAGNOSTICS REPORT
       REF. RANGE:     SCANNED IN EPIC

      W20574 COLL: 01/29/2014 11:52 REC: 01/29/2014 11:57 PHYS: FLYNN, PATRICK MICHAEL

      CORTISOL
```

PROGESTERONE	0.00	ng/mL

```
    PROGESTERONE           0.00                     ng/mL
                    Female Progesterone Reference Range:
                      Ovulatory Cycle:
                        Follicular:    0.15- 1.40 ng/mL
                        Luteal:        3.34-25.56 ng/mL
                        Midluteal:     4.44-28.03 ng/mL
                        Postmenopausal: <0.21-0.73 ng/mL

                    Pregnant Female Progesterone Ref. Ranges:
                      First Trimester:   11.22- 90.00 ng/mL
                      Second Trimester:  25.55- 89.40 ng/mL
                      Third Trimester:   48.40-422.50 ng/mL

    T3, TOTAL              0.75              [0.60-1.90] ng/mL

    T4, TOTAL             11.2              [4.8-13.9] ug/dL

    TESTOSTERONE        L 7.3               [14.0-76.0] ng/dL

    TSH                  2.820             [0.358-3.740] uIU/mL

    DHEA SULFATE:        <15
                         Reference range: < OR = 145
                         Unit: mcg/dL
                         (NOTE)
             Test Performed at:
             Quest Diagnostics Nichols Institute
             33608 Ortega Highway
             San Juan Capistrano, CA  92675-2042      J M Nakamoto MD, PhD

    TBG ASSESSMENT:       1.12
                         Reference range: 0.79 to 1.16
                         (NOTE)
             Test Performed at:
             Quest Diagnostics Nichols Institute
             33608 Ortega Highway
             San Juan Capistrano, CA  92675-2042      J M Nakamoto MD, PhD

       PATIENT:                              Print Date-Time: 02/11/2014 -15:04
                              PATIENT REPORT
```

have her do and since they hadn't found anything, they put her on a psychiatric drug. They did what they knew, but I asked her if they had ever tested her hormones. The answer was no.

I started with the proper hormone testing. Come to find out, her progesterone levels were at zero. She sat with me and her son and as we were going over her tests and she started crying. She said three words, "I'm not crazy." Don't confuse hormonal problems with psychiatric problems.

Don't confuse hormonal problems with psychiatric problems.

There could be something more going on. I wonder how many women will spend their whole lives thinking they are crazy like this poor woman did. I'm frustrated and I'm not even one of these women! That woman was seventy, let's look at the other end of the spectrum.

Before I tell this story, I want to assure you I'm sharing this information with your best interest at heart. I have four daughters, and I have to deal with this personally. Be very careful letting your young daughters play sports. Not that they are incapable, but if they get heavily involved and are consistently doing high levels of physical activity, they can harm their hormone levels. Knowing what we know about female hormones, you can see the problems this can mean for them. Boys are very different—a good way of building testosterone is moving and

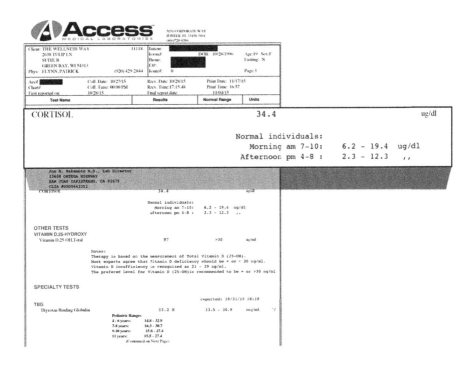

exercise. Protect your young girls from the kind of physical exercise that will drain their hormones very quickly.

This nineteen-year-old woman is a runner and a Division 1 scholarship winner for track and field. Do you know what happens to women runners' cycles? They lose them. It's common, but common does not mean normal. The school told her if she didn't run, they'd pull her scholarship. So, as a result, she's physically stressed, mentally stressed and lost her cycle. Why? When you rev the engine really high and don't know how to fuel it, you're going to lose your normal physiology. We tested her stress hormone. It was so high, it was

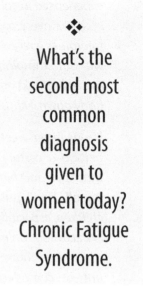

What's the second most common diagnosis given to women today? Chronic Fatigue Syndrome.

double off the chart even at the chart's highest value. Yes, you can test stress hormone. It's called cortisol. Remember, hormones are high in the morning and lower at night. If the levels are very high all the time, it's chronic stress. If the levels go very low and they empty out, you experience fatigue. What's the second most common diagnosis given to women today? Chronic Fatigue Syndrome. Let me guess how many of you have had your cortisol tested. Your stress hormones can actually tell your doctor where your body is functioning; high stress or fatigue. The whole key is this, we don't test for fires, we test for function. It's very important to get your stress hormones tested, especially if you are a woman. How we take care of you differs as those hormones fluctuate.

CHRISTY'S THOUGHTS

> *I agree that sports can be detrimental to a young woman's health… that's why testing and knowledge about hormones and how to become and stay healthy is so crucial. But I would add that it doesn't have to be sports…college itself can be stressful. The stress that I*

experienced in college was depleting my hormones to the point that I felt like every organ in my body was shutting down. From having migraines every day for an entire semester, to not being able to eat without cramping or becoming ill, to having periodic chest pains, anxiety attacks and female issues. Stress was successfully shutting my body down. I chose to lessen my stress load by changing my major.

It was bittersweet, but my health was more important to me than getting a certain degree. What I didn't realize at that time was that God had bigger plans for me than the small plans I had for myself. Don't put unreasonable expectations on yourself or your children, especially if they are female. I was the one who put the high expectations on myself, and I suffered as a result. I wish I had known more about hormone health back then. You can't change the past, but you can affect the future. I will definitely be advocating for my children so that we can enjoy grandchildren someday!!

Some women tell me they are more of a night person than a morning person. That may seem harmless enough, but it's actually an indicator that you are sick. Hormones, and correspondingly energy, are supposed to be highest in the morning. If you have a hard time getting through the morning and at night when you are not supposed to have much hormone, you feel you can take on the world, your rhythms are off. You are supposed to rest at night. Most people have too much hormone at night and not enough during the day. That's why we ask patients if they are night people or morning people—it's a great clue for us. If their hormones aren't getting high enough at the proper times, that's why they struggle to get their bodies out of bed. At night when you don't need as much, every little bit feels like enough to keep powering through. Now this is a tough one, because most women say they feel fine. They report having a hard time getting out of bed and better able to get a lot done at night. They don't want us to mess up that energy! I understand that, but health needs to come first.

If all of these changes happen as the month goes on, and it doesn't go right, that last zone can be unknown. You don't know who you are walking into that day. But if you take the advice I give you, make sure she is tested properly, and help that woman through her cycle, you'll enter the Bonus Zone! This is when libido soars and she becomes just like you again. If her hormones have not been properly supported up until this point, then it's back to the Woman Zone. How's that for motivation to help your wife out?

Zone 4: The Bonus Zone

Ladies, let me give you a little mental peace. Honestly, you should only have a sex drive about two weeks of the month. Let me say that again. Physiologically you should only have a sex drive two weeks of the month. If you have a sex drive all month long, you are sick and better get checked out. Your husband will be happy, but your hormones have become very abnormal and you're going to end up with some health conditions.

This final week is the week that will let you know how you did the first three weeks of the month. We either have another Man Zone or another Woman Zone. I think we can all agree which we'd prefer—healthy hormones!

ZONE 4
UNKNOWN ZONE

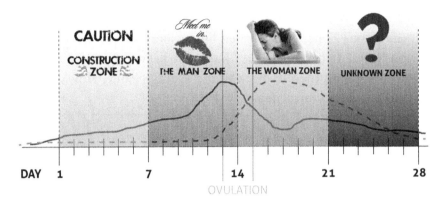

KEY　— ESTRADIOL　- - - PROGESTERONE

ZONE 4
BONUS ZONE

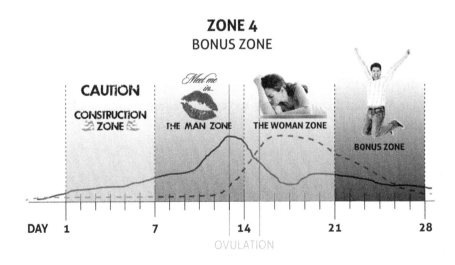

KEY　— ESTRADIOL　- - - PROGESTERONE

Okay guys, here's your second To Do List.

#1 Help the Girl.

I don't just believe this, I know this. It's very difficult to have a woman's body—they have a lot going on. They change every week. They don't always understand this, so they think there is something wrong with them. Ladies, there's nothing wrong, it's what your body does. Help her to know she is not crazy, she is normal. Help her deal with stress and life. Help her make wise food choices. Help her.

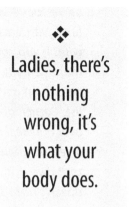

Ladies, there's nothing wrong, it's what your body does.

Christy's Thoughts:

I know that there is a very large feminist movement of women who want to 'do everything a man can', but I disagree! Women have become so sick as a result of this faulty thinking. Our bodies were not meant to take on that much stress. And there is nothing wrong with that. It doesn't mean that women are not capable or can't have certain positions or roles in companies. After all, our two top CEO's in our companies are women. But my husband and I understand how much stress they can handle, and he is committed to teaching all of our staff and their spouses about setting priorities and making sure to use time management effectively in accomplishing their priorities. We women can do one thing a man CAN'T, and that is bear children. God created us to be able to have children, and, in my opinion, it is an amazing gift that should not be treated lightly. There are so many women, just like me, who have been lied to and told that they cannot have children. I disagree!

Recently I lost my mother. Patrick, knowing that my family is on my priority list, was able to help me to spend the time I needed with my family. Patrick was able to take on more responsibility that I normally took care of at home so that I could be with my Dad and siblings as we dealt with funeral arrangements and spent much-needed time with each other. That's what Patrick means by 'helping your wife'. If you can successfully fulfill your priorities with effective time management, you can insert yourself into your spouse's schedule to help them accomplish what they need to get done on their priority list. Patrick does this all the time! I don't expect it though. We talk over our weekly schedules on Sundays, and then, if he is able, he can insert his ability to help me. Now ladies, I feel like I do need to mention that if your husband is offering to help you, and it's something that doesn't need specific instruction, please let him do it HIS way. Like doing the dishes or cleaning, or getting the kids ready for school or bed—if he is offering to do it, girl, you need to step aside and let him do it!! Likewise, if he is offering to do something that would actually cause you more stress, just simply thank him and politely decline, but offer something else that he can do to help you. Ladies, if he wants to help you, you need to let him help you, and, although he may think he is Superman, he cannot read your mind.

#2 DON'T STRESS THE GIRL.

You can be the greatest thing to help her be healthy, or the biggest factor in making her sick. Please don't be that kind of guy. It's really sad, but guys don't understand this, and neither do women. Let me give you an example of a situation I had in San Francisco. I was speaking and a woman who considered herself a feminist came up to me and said "Doctor, I disagree. I can handle just as much stress as a man." I asked her why she was there. She said, "Because I'm sick." I told her, "Take a seat, I think you may be surprised at what you learn today." I wasn't being disrespectful, but understand your body doesn't function based on your beliefs. You don't have to believe me—the research has been done, and you can find it in books as well as online. Mental stress will drain your hormones. Physical stress will drain your hormones. Chemicals will drain your hormones. Guys are lucky in that stress does not affect our hormones. The guy can have a horrible day. Work was challenging, the kids' behavior sucked, and still he gets home at night and what does he want? SEX. A lady has stress, and guys, you know there's very little chance of visiting the Man Cave that night. Right? Why? It changes their body when they stress out. Ladies, you may not want to hear this, but take comfort in it: you are not designed to handle stress like a man, your biology will never let you. Men, it's your job to reduce the stress of a woman. This alone should relieve stress for women.

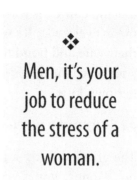

Men, it's your job to reduce the stress of a woman.

#3 PROTECT THE GIRL

I got home one day, and I could tell right away that my wife and daughter were not having a good time. Christy told me, "Go talk to your daughter!"

So, I took Faith to our favorite organic tea spot and after a little chatting she starts "Daddy…"

I interrupted her, "Whoa, whoa, whoa, before you say anything, remember this, that's my wife. I will protect my wife from anybody, including you. So, when you go home, you're going to go and apologize to your mother. Remember, if you make her stressed out, you can make her sick. You are eventually going to grow up and leave her, I'm not."

After a while, we went home, and they talked. I still to this day don't even know what the problem was. The next morning when I went to wake Faith, she said, "Daddy, before you go, I just want to say I'm sorry for making Mom mad last night."

I told her, "Don't worry, God forgives, just move on." She went on to say, "Daddy, I've been thinking about it a lot. I know why I drive Mom so crazy."

"Really, you do?"

"Yeah, I'm just like you!" I laughed like crazy. Oh my goodness—where did she come up with that?! Christy would tell you she's the image of me in every way. It's worth noting: when men get stressed, they'll leave their wife and bond to their kids. Be aware and don't do that. Bond to your wife. She needs you two to stay connected. Protect her, even from her own kids.

#4 SCHEDULE WITH THE GIRL

The greatest thing a guy could say to his wife in the morning would be, "Honey, would you like to go on a date with me?" Oh guys, if you could only see the room full of smiling ladies I see when I say this in one of my seminars. Guys, when you first met that woman, you did everything. Your testosterone was driven, you created pictures in your mind, you chased her, you dated her, and you scheduled things with her. She's still the same way, but most guys have stopped doing those things. Her biology will always desire to connect with you. One of the best things guys can do is to continue to date their wives. If you do this, and you plan it, she'll create the picture in her mind of all the wonderful things that make you to be the most amazing man in her world. I still date my wife! I plan it all, including the dance classes that I recently signed us up for. I told her in advance, and she was so excited before our date and beaming after our date. My wife likes dancing, you will have to think about what your wife likes. It doesn't have to be fancy if you show her that you see her and understand her. Guys, how much does that cost you? A little effort perhaps, but it pays off huge. Plan it. You plan it, guys. When you were first chasing her and pursuing her, you planned everything. Then when you married her, it becomes, "What do you want to do?"

One of the best things guys can do is to continue to date their wives.

Don't do that. You plan it, that connects with her. Take her somewhere peaceful to sit and just ask her, "Honey, how was your day?" That gives a woman the opportunity to talk for the next three-and-a-half hours and you don't have to do anything. I'm kidding! But when she talks, she's connecting. What does that do to her hormones? It makes her healthy. Think about that. It's very simple.

Now I hear, "Doc, we do all of these things and my wife still doesn't respond."

#5 Test the Girl

Today, women deal with more hormonal problems than ever in history and they are as sick as can be. It's why we have more fertility problems and more cancers. This concept we started nineteen years ago has become a national brand for this reason. It's a different thought process that's easy to apply with a doctor that does things from this perspective. When we apply this different process to patients, we get different results— results completely different from what the traditional medicine approach can achieve. Right now, based on medical statistics, heart disease rates are going up and cancer rates are going up. If you don't change your

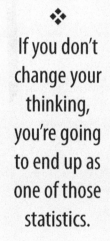

❖
If you don't change your thinking, you're going to end up as one of those statistics.

thinking, you're going to end up as one of those statistics. My wife could have been one of those statistics. This is very real. Remember, don't accept common for normal.

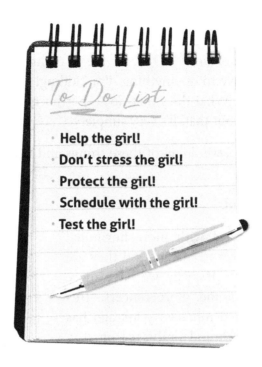

Joy's Story

I had been a healthy young woman until I went off the Depo-Provera injections I was using as birth control. The years leading up to our Wellness Way journey had been filled with tons of attempts to finding natural remedies to balance my hormones and tons of frustration and disappointment with each one. I was almost 30-years-old. My husband and I had been married for 10 years. By this time, we had a miscarriage and lost twins. I was heartbroken and losing hope of having children.

To top things off, I had just had my adrenal function tested and was told I'd be on medication for the rest of my life.

From the moment we walked into The Wellness Way and our first appointment with Dr. Patrick, things were different. He was so upbeat and positive, even after we shared the adrenal test results with him. This was the first time I'd ever seen a doctor upbeat or positive after looking at my situation. To be honest, this was what gave me hope to continue on. In fact, during our first appointment he said, "Give me six months, and you'll be pregnant!" How could I not have hope?

Well, sure enough, we had our first baby girl in 2009! We were so excited when we conceived our first miracle. You can only imagine our surprise and amazement when three months later we conceived our second baby girl! Fifteen months after our second daughter was born, we conceived our son.

Not only was Dr. Patrick invaluable in helping us start our family, but with two babies so close together, and a third shortly after you can only imagine all the hormone fluctuations. He was an amazing help through the breastfeeding, post-partum care and nearly back to back pregnancies. And those adrenals? No problem.

One thing I can say about Dr. Patrick, when he gets your hormones where they need to be, they work just fine!

CHAPTER 10

No Control with Birth Control

This happens every day, imagine the day in the life of an average couple. Jill looks up briefly as her husband, Bob, gets home and returns to scrubbing the counter. As he walks in Bob senses something isn't right. He asks, "Jill, is something wrong?" She looks up exasperated. He doesn't know what to do, so he moves to hug her. As soon as he touches her, Jill gets so frustrated she wants to scream, but she doesn't know why, so instead she starts to cry. She shakes uncontrollably as she cries and pushes him away. Neither of them connects it right away to the birth control pill Jill recently started taking. It sounds dramatic, but I have heard stories like this many times before.

Many women don't connect their hormone problems and other ailments to this common endocrine disruptor. Nearly 80% of women between the ages of fifteen and forty-four have used the birth control pill at some point in their lives. Very few of those women have taken out their magnifying glass to look at the insert that comes with that monthly prescription of birth control pills. If they did, they would see a long list of side effects.

Some of the Potential Risks, Side Effects and Adverse Reactions Listed in the Insert:

- Risk of developing blood clots
- Heart attacks and strokes
- Gall bladder disease
- Liver tumors
- Cancer of the reproductive organs and breasts
- Irregular vaginal bleeding
- Changes in vision
- Melasma
- Change in appetite
- Nausea
- Headache
- Nervousness
- Mental Depression
- Dizziness
- Loss of scalp hair
- Rash
- Vaginal infections
- Allergic reactions
- Gastrointestinal Symptoms
- Weight gain
- Vaginal candidiasis
- Pre-menstrual syndrome
- Acne
- Changes in libido

If you can't tell from the list-don't mess with the female body, the balance is so delicate. The minute you disrupt one hormone in a female's body, it sets off a cascade of many bad side effects.

Birth control itself is an endocrine disruptor. It disrupts your hormones which will disrupt all of the systems like the gears in the Swiss watch. When you start taking birth control pills you are giving your body synthetic hormones, so your body stops making them itself. This means your hormones are controlled synthetically, and the body's production of hormones goes to menopausal levels. This doesn't help your body function. It <u>keeps</u> your body from normal function. This sets your body up for problems now and even more problems down the road. It sets you up to be very sick.

> ❖
> **When you start taking birth control pills you are giving your body synthetic hormones, so your body stops making them itself.**

Birth control hormones disrupt your whole system. They alter your whole endocrine system and your endocrine system determines your life. When you were a young lady and started your cycle, your genes did not change, your habits did not change—your hormones changed. It changed your whole body, including your thinking, and now you're going to take a disruptor. Knowing what you now know about female hormones, do you really think it's going to be okay?

It's not. We have come as a country to think hormonal birth control is harmless. Sometimes we are even told it's beneficial! I'm telling you now, it's neither harmless nor beneficial. I wish they were. These prescriptions cause a host of complications like infertility, cancer, hormone imbalance, and low libido. The convenience they offer is surely not worth the damage. No, it's not a popular stance to take, but it's an important one. The conditions that are the terrible consequences of these drugs are on the rise, and often the damage is irreversible. I will continue to share the truth until we see all these conditions start a pattern of decline. We need to stop sacrificing the health of women for convenience.

The couple from our scenario, Jill and Bob decided that Jill would go on birth control to prevent pregnancy until they were ready to have kids. This is a decision many couples make. The pill was the option they chose so they could have sex without worrying about pregnancy. Ironically, they have started a new cascade of worries. How intimate can a couple get if her hormones are out of balance? Intimacy is typically the last thing a woman is interested in if they have gained weight, have headaches, depression, vaginal infections or any other side effects.

When they are ready to have that baby, will her body be ready? Her hormones have been disrupted for so long, we don't know what they will be like. They might find her hormones don't just come back after she stops taking the pill. When Jill and Bob want to have kids, they may run into fertility problems. Then we will have to work on rebuilding Jill's hormones. It could take lots of heartbreak and unnecessary spending to rebuild hormones because her hormonal balance was destroyed by this endocrine disruptor. Not everyone is lucky enough to rebuild them.

Some women do everything in their routine naturally, but then they take birth control because their husband wants them to. I wonder if they would be so eager if they knew the health disruptions of increased cervical cancer rates and increased breast

Who says there are increased rates of breast and cervical cancer? "They" do! Read the inserts.

cancer rates. Who says there are increased rates of breast and cervical cancer? "They" do! Read the inserts.

Each week, I do a live recording of "The Dr. Patrick Flynn Show." Viewers and patients send us questions, so we can respond live and unscripted. It's a great outlet for many questions to be answered while getting the right information to people seeking answers. Here's a question and then I will give you my response from one episode.

> *Hi Dr. Patrick, I am thirty-two years old. We have three children; my husband does not want anymore but I would not mind. He wants me on birth control. I started taking it and I don't feel good; I don't even feel like the same person! I've gained weight, I'm more emotional, but my husband said he will NOT use condoms. I've been following you for a long time and know it's not good for me and the more I research I do, I'm scared that I'm taking it. What research can I give him to convince him that I should not be on it? Also, he says it is fine because my OB said it was the best way to prevent another pregnancy.*

First, we'll take this from the relationship side. Ladies, this is an interesting situation. Women will take care of their bodies. However, if their husband suggests for them to do something different, they will frequently, quickly, do it. Typically, this is due to the deep need for connection and their desire to keep the peace in the relationship. You want research to convince him birth control is bad for you? Stop having sex with him. There's your research. Ok, that sounds aggressive, but hang in there with me. The research is everywhere. It's even on the package insert. His concern should be your health, not his convenience the few days a month you may be fertile. Unless

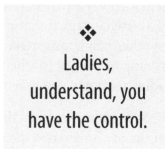

❖

Ladies, understand, you have the control.

he uses condoms, you aren't having sex. Ladies, understand, you have the control.

I know I'll hear from Christian ladies out there, "But Doc, being a Christian woman, I just have to do what he wants and submit." My friend Ross Allen Skorzewski, who is my host on "The Dr. Patrick Flynn Show," has worked in the church for over twenty years and has plenty of experience in marriage and relationship counseling. He has also worked with some of the greatest marriage enrichments speakers around the world. Here's his response to this argument:

> *Stop over-spiritualizing this situation. If he is putting you in an unhealthy place, and now we are talking about birth control, you need to look at this more clearly. He says he won't use condoms. The only option for him to be intimate with you is for you to put this unhealthy poison into your body. You need to rattle that boy's cage. You need to get a hold of him and shut down the shop and say, "The Man Cave is closed." This isn't about submitting, this is about dysfunction junction. He needs to look at his relationship with his wife and not just his own needs. He may just want sex now, but he'll be getting a lot less of that as his wife's body gets sicker. The dysfunction has to stop. This has to be about a healthy relationship and healthy bodies, together.*

According to the email, it doesn't even look like it was a discussion, and often it's not. He may have said he won't use condoms and she needs to take birth control. Because she desires that relationship, she caves. On the other hand, testosterone is a powerful motivator. If condoms are his only way to get to where he wants to go, he'll soon happily oblige. Ladies, trust me, you have more control over him than you think.

Here's another angle to this, the OB said it was the best thing for her to use to *prevent pregnancy*. It doesn't mean it's best for her body. Technically, there is an even better way to prevent pregnancy.

Abstinence. You'll have no kids if there is no sex. Frustrating? Sure, but you won't have to worry about pregnancy! It sounds silly and extreme, but honestly, the moment you tell him no, he'll go for a while without being intimate with you, but he'll quickly consider the use of condoms.

Looking at it from a health standpoint. Birth control is very detrimental to female health. It is an endocrine disrupter as defined by the EPA. It throws off the cycle and trust me, you'll end up with problems. The woman who sent the email was looking for help because she did break down and take the birth control. She knew right away she was starting to feel sick. Picture this. If the average person who has no medical conditions then takes a medication, it makes them sick. Remember what medication does? It forces a response. Actually, medication by pharmacology definition is a non-lethal dose of a lethal substance. If a healthy person takes a medication,

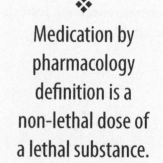

❖
Medication by pharmacology definition is a non-lethal dose of a lethal substance.

they become sick. This woman has three beautiful kids and apparently no problems with pregnancies and now goes on a hormone disruptor. She's going to feel sick.

This woman now doesn't feel like the same vibrant person she was before the birth control. Every time she looks at herself, she's probably bothered by the weight gain and her emotions are completely off. She's not going to be interested in sex. She's going to shut down because of all the changes going on in her body. Women, you are so self-conscious about your bodies. Most guys don't care about the subtle changes like weight gain in your body. But for you, this is huge and will disrupt your whole being, including your long-term health. Keep your best interests at heart, and say no to prescription birth control. If he becomes disrespectful and disruptive, my heart goes out to you for the kind of man you are dealing with. However, he doesn't control you, especially if it means causing you health problems.

I would hope that men would have their wives' best interest in mind; her health and physiology, her emotions, their relationship and even his own health. Because if they understood what birth control does, they wouldn't ask their ladies to put this into their bodies. Men, part of protecting her is protecting her health. If she thinks you'll stop loving her if she says no to prescription birth control, it's time for some serious reflection. Testosterone makes you great at protection—don't be afraid to use it.

Ladies if you are on birth control, every time you kiss him or you have sex with him, he gets the hormone.

Here's something few people realize about prescriptions, including birth control: that hormone shows up in your bodily fluids, not just your bloodstream. It is also in your saliva and your vaginal secretions. Ladies if you are on birth control, every time you kiss him or you have sex with him, he gets the hormone. You are passing it to him. I have men come into the office and their estrogen and progesterone levels are way off. They ask me how it's possible. Is your wife on birth control? Well, then you're taking it too. When men realize this, and understand these synthetic hormones are also affecting his body and will create problems for him as well, they're quick to reconsider their stance on the matter!

One of the number one side effects of birth control? Cancer. Remember that insert of info from the pill packet. That will list all the disruptions it will cause in the woman's body, including cancer.

Sex without condoms becomes much less of a concern if and when a family is devastated by cancer.

Pills are not the only form of prescription birth control capable of causing such problems with hormones and health. IUDs and the patch are just a disruptive. You are not safe if you are using another endocrine disrupter form of birth control like the hormonal IUD, vaginal ring, implants or the patch; all these things are destructive to hormones. Fortunately, there are non-hormonal options.

There are other natural methods to prevent pregnancy:

- Diaphragm
- Condoms
- Family planning

Not all women who are on birth control are taking it to prevent pregnancy. A study found 14% of women are taking the pill for non-contraceptive reasons. Many more relied on it for non-contraceptive purposes in addition to contraception with only 42% using it exclusively for contraception. I wonder if the numbers would be the same if they all knew the consequences.

CHRISTY'S THOUGHTS

I was grateful when my mother told me that because of her own reproductive issues, she was not going to encourage us to get 'the pill' or any other drugs that doctors claimed would help. Even though my cystic acne was so bad, I got good at covering it up and many times avoided staying the night at friends' houses to avoid the embarrassment of them seeing me without it. Even though I got migraines in college that were just the beginning of a seemingly downhill spiral of a hormone imbalance caused by stress was slowly taking over my life. Even back then, I just refused to believe that everything could be fixed with 'the pill'. Then came the cysts and the incredible pain...and the only solution medical doctors had was drugs and surgery. Well, I'm so glad that I disagreed before I even knew better. Had I continued to go down the road they were recommending, I would not have had our four amazing girls!

Pharmaceutical companies are very good at marketing their products for a multitude of purposes, and birth control is no exception. They use what they know to address all kinds of concerns: acne, heavy periods, polycystic ovarian syndrome, endometriosis, migraines, and more. Each of those is regularly treated with a type of prescription birth control. You'll notice something interesting when you look at the inserts to see the potential negative effects. Some of them are the *very ones* they are treating you for.

You shouldn't have bad acne, horrible periods, or cysts and all that can come from imbalanced hormones. If your hormones are out of control, it's not because you aren't taking a birth control pill. It's because your hormones are off balance. You can take all the medication you want to, but it doesn't fix the underlying problem. Thinking differently, getting your hormones tested and knowing how to best support your body to bring them back into balance will bring you clinical results pills can't.

You can take all the medication you want to, but it doesn't fix the underlying problem.

A study followed women in Denmark for ten years and found those women taking hormonal contraception had a 40% higher rate of developing depression. For young women, birth control pills are even gloomier. Those who were between the ages of fifteen and nineteen taking combination birth control pills, were diagnosed with depression at a rate seventy percent higher than those who weren't taking the pill. Another study tracked half a million women and found that the risk of attempting suicide <u>doubled</u> for those taking hormonal birth control!

When we look at the risks and the impacts on hormonal balance, it's much bigger than just preventing pregnancy, or treating another condition. Prescription birth control is actually *causing* conditions we are working feverishly to stop! What's the easiest way to stop a condition though? Taking a different path—one that won't harm you to begin with.

Chapter 11

Puberty Comes Too Soon

Imagine a young girl visiting my office with her mom. Her feet swing underneath her chair as she reads a book, so the seven-year-old doesn't seem to hear us talking about precocious puberty—puberty at an early age. Her mom looks at me nervously as we sit in my office. Not only is this mom's niece experiencing this "normal phenomenon" of boobs at age eight, but she hears other moms at the playground talking about it too. Someone told her it was because of the meat they ate; another person said it was because of the milk. Mom looks at me with a panicked look that I have seen a lot lately from patients who have children, "Do I have to worry about my second grader and puberty? Isn't that something for middle school and high school? Is this normal?"

Having daughters, I get extremely serious about this. No, it's not normal, but we have been seeing the first signs of puberty is happening younger. It's now eight and nine-year-olds. Sometimes it's even kindergartners or younger. Who wants to be teaching their kindergartner about bras and how to tie their shoes? Not me. That comes fast enough.

If you go back in history, even fifty years ago, the average start of menstruation was between fifteen and sixteen years old. If you look at Biblical times, the Bible is such great documentation of history, most people were married and sometimes having kids right after menstruation began. Could you imagine if your daughter had her cycle at ten years old? Go back in history and with menstruation starting at fifteen, sixteen or even seventeen, these young women were almost adults already. What has been the change that has happened to cause early development?

What used to be late teens, and a signal it was time to be married, is happening too soon. Eight years old is too soon. Who would be ready to marry off their eight-year-old? I want more time for tea parties and doll houses. Over the past century, the age of first period has gone down worldwide from sixteen to under age thirteen. We are also seeing increased incidents of precocious puberty. This is when very young girls are experiencing puberty outside the normal window. What causes early puberty?

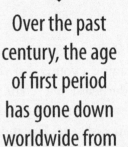

Over the past century, the age of first period has gone down worldwide from sixteen to under age thirteen.

Our genome has not changed. A common thought is that this is controlled by genetics; however, that's not the case. The purpose of genetics is to keep your body normal, to support life. When you are born your genes make sure you develop to a healthy and normal state. If there is disruption during development, you can see some changes, but genes are not the determining factor here.

What causes puberty? What changes for girls that doesn't happen to boys? Estrogen levels go up for girls and this leads to many of the changes that girls see when they enter puberty. Girls are ten times more likely to experience central precocious puberty. Also, when girls are diagnosed, they do not know the cause, whereas with boys they are able to identify an underlying cause.

So, what's the cause? As we've learned, females are complicated, and so is our modern environment. As such, there are several contributing factors, rather than just one. The only thing that causes you to go from child to young adulthood is estrogen levels starting to rise. Estrogens can come from any number of places, including food and environment. If they are forced synthetically (prescriptions) or introduced to your body through other means, your gene system will respond to that environment. Once you have induced puberty though, there is no going back.

What do you want to avoid? What in our environment is leading to estrogen levels increasing? We see the impacts of increased estrogens easily on young girls, but the same increased levels of estrogen are impacting us all. Making changes for our daughters is important, but we also want to make them for ourselves. The meat and hormone issues are very well known and well documented—we'll look at that first.

They put the hormones into the cow to increase the growth rate and the mass of that animal. If you go back 200-300 years ago, the only people who ate muscle meat were the peasants, the slaves, and people of lower social statuses. Organ meats were the delicacy. The king wouldn't eat a muscle meat, that's peasant meat. What changed? If you talk to a young person about an organ meat, they freak out. Years ago, Grandma's house had liver paste. She happily served it, and we happily sat there eating heart, liver, kidney, and tongue. The shift came when the farming industry recognized they couldn't increase production of organs at a high rate, but they *could* increase muscle meat. Now instead of grass feeding livestock, we're grain feeding them, which makes them grow bigger and faster. The food industry has come to value speed, convenience, and quantity. This is as a result of a number of influences, but the clear result is a clear decline in quality. I get people who say,

"Doc, healthy food is so expensive." Now that's opening the door to an entirely new conversation, but the question I usually ask then is: "Do you ever wonder why other food can be so cheap?" Most of it something closer to a food-like product, not food.

The industry has focused on getting the animal to be larger, to weigh more so they can sell more as quickly as possible. This makes sense for them as a business—more product equals more sales! I understand! But the other side of the conversation is this: if you ingest the synthetic hormones added to meat, you're going to alter your hormones. Growth hormones in meat are causing women's estrogens to go up higher than they are supposed to and it's inducing faster maturity and puberty. So yes, meat can do it, but it's not the only thing. Let's be clear, I am not saying to quit eating meat. I'm saying get a good source. Ask a local organic farmer what they feed their cows and buy half a cow. It's cheaper, healthier, and supports local industry!

❖

The number one source of hormone introduction to the human body comes from city water.

There are many other triggers of precocious puberty. Meat is just one. If there is an introduction of hormones into *any* food source, it can induce early maturation and puberty. Do you know what the number one source for everyone—male, female, and child—to come in contact with hormones? It's not meats. The number one source of hormone introduction to the human body comes from city water.

Not long ago, I went up to see my sister in Spokane, Washington. We went to the gorgeous river. Right next to it was a water treatment facility. They're sucking the water and cleaning it out and pushing it back into the system. When we drove by, I pointed out to my sister that there's no filtration. Well, there's filtration, but here's what's happening. Water is treated for mineral content—anything that is naturally occurring in nature is treated and filtered in the plant. Things like Sulphur and Iron. If you've ever been somewhere with high Sulphur in the water, you appreciate how great that filtration is! What's not filtered however, are chemicals. When a woman who takes birth control pills pees, it goes into the water system and gets recycled back. Water treatment facilities don't have the type of filtration necessary to get prescription drugs back out of the system. With the increasing number of prescription drugs getting flushed into the system, this is a growing issue. At a municipal level, getting the filtration in place to address this is cost-prohibitive to say the least. However, you can easily add filtration to your home! The alternative, if you do not have proper water filtration on your house, is that you are exposed to everyone else's synthetic hormones in your showers, your cooking, and your drinking water.

Meat and water are two major contributors to early puberty. There are many other things considered endocrine disruptors that will also raise the estrogens levels in young girls. Many of them we come into contact with daily. The heavy metals in dental fillings, plastic water bottles and food storage, soft plastic toys and vinyl, metal cans for canned food, household cleaners and fragrances, flame retardants on children's pajamas and other household products all contain endocrine disruptors that change reproductive hormones.

There is one more "healthy food" that needs to be addressed. Soy. Soy contains phytoestrogens. These are plant-based compounds that mimic human hormones. Soy is very prevalent in our processed foods today. It is used in so many ways throughout the food industry that you are still most likely getting soy even when you don't realize it. Then there are the "health" advocates who say they are avoiding meats but turn to soy as a protein source. They are no better off on the hormone issue than those eating meat.

Here's an interesting one—one that seems indirect but isn't. You know what else can impact the onset of puberty? Whether your child plays outside or not. Children who are inside all the time playing video games or watching T.V. are more often less physically active. Physical activity is key to preventing obesity. According to the CDC, 17.4% of children ages six to eleven are obese. This is important because estrogen is stored in fat. Studies have shown, girls who are obese will get their first period a year earlier than those who are not. Overweight boys will also see earlier signs of puberty, but studies have shown obese boys will have later start of puberty which could be because of greater estrogen production in the obese boys.

Another reason to get your kids outside—they need vitamin D. Vitamin D is a vital hormone to keep the body functioning optimally. Studies have shown a link between vitamin D deficiency and early puberty. Girls closer to the equator will have a later start than those further away who don't see the sun as much. That's not good. One study showed girls who were vitamin D deficient were twice as likely to get their period early than those who had plenty of vitamin D.

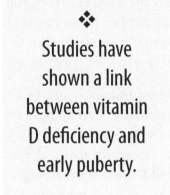

❖

Studies have shown a link between vitamin D deficiency and early puberty.

There are multiple things that can drive up estrogen levels. Remember, the body is like a Swiss watch. Like we have talked about, the only thing to cause the change from child to young womanhood are those estrogen levels coming up. If they are forced artificially, your gene system will respond to the environment and bring on puberty. There is no reversing this effect.

So yes, we are looking at this issue of breasts getting bigger and earlier in girls. There are a number of things we can do to address this. The mother was right that the meat source is possibly one of the causes due to the hormones that have been injected into that animal. That is a simple change—meat without hormones is becoming more and more readily available as we learn the impact of those synthetics. Some of the other exposures to hormones through the diet may need to be addressed. Does she need to worry because they are related? No, this is not a genetic issue. Your genes respond to help you to live the longest and healthiest life possible. You are not genetically programmed to suffer or be sick.

You are not genetically programmed to suffer or be sick.

It seems like a lot. There are a variety of triggers. We can't blame one thing or take a pill to get our desired outcome. But I'm excited to share this information with you, because there are so many things you CAN do. There is a lot we can control if we take the time. We can clean it up—starting at home. Then in our communities—for our daughters and ourselves. Estrogens effect boys and adults too.

It's worth the time. Time is precious especially when it's time to be a kid. As the father of four girls, I know it goes fast. They deserve this time to swing their legs under their chair and not worry about our conversations about puberty. It all comes soon enough.

CHAPTER 12

The "M" Word

Menopause is a bad word for many women. Most women cringe and fear the experience even before they enter this natural process. There aren't many women throwing parties for this transition in their life. But what if I told you women do not have to experience the difficult "symptoms" that menopause can cause? First, let's understand what menopause is and what it isn't.

When you say the word menopause to a woman, do they think healthy, vital and sexual right away? No. They think vaginal dryness, period problems, night sweats. That's not menopause. If you have any of these problems, I'll agree they're common, but with the new way of thinking we're learning in this book, I want to show you that these symptoms are actually a sign you are sick. Menopause doesn't have to be that way.

Standard medical thinking and approach treats menopause like an unavoidable syndrome for women. The inevitable monster that is bound to rough you up any time after fifty years old. Its waiting for you, and it's just the way it is. It's exclusive to women, and very different from anything a man

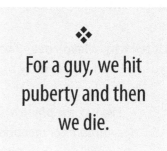

For a guy, we hit puberty and then we die.

experiences. For a guy, we hit puberty and then we die. That's about it; if we keep ourselves healthy.

The largest medical establishment in the country is Mayo Clinic. Mayo defines menopause perfectly, but let me use their definition to show you the incongruent thinking.

Here's the Mayo Clinic definition:

> *Menopause is defined as occurring 12 months after your last menstrual period and marks the end of the menstrual cycles. Menopause can happen in your 40s or 50s with the average American woman beginning at age 51.*

Ladies, if you go through menopause in your forties, that's alright, just get your hormone levels tested to be sure that is what is really happening. So far we're doing great with this definition.

> *Menopause is a natural biological process. Although it also ends fertility, you can stay healthy, vital and sexual. Some women feel relieved because they no longer worry about pregnancy.*

They're correct. Everything Mayo Clinic said to that point is perfect. But there's a disconnect. If I were to walk up to a woman and tell her, "Menopause keeps you healthy, vital and sexual," they'd look at me, laugh, and ask, "What planet are you from?"

Here's why. Mayo's next paragraph, after that perfect definition, is what women actually identify menopause with.

> *Even so, the physical symptoms such as hot flashes, and emotional symptoms of menopause may disrupt your sleep, lower energy and for some women trigger anxiety and feelings of sadness and loss.*

This is where the confusion comes in. How can you be healthy, vital and sexual with that list of symptoms? This is where traditional medicine is limited in their perspective. Everything they've been taught—and therefore teach—is correct, but what they don't have is the thinking that would allow them to support hormone levels and *prevent* those symptoms. Menopause is a natural biological state and process, but it doesn't have to be miserable or medicated. Recently, Mayo updated their definition—sadly, they removed the part about staying healthy, vital, and sexual.

I had a sixty-four-year-old woman come in to see me. Her primary complaint was how she was suffering so badly from menopause symptoms. Guess what my first question was. Have you ever had your hormones tested? I wanted her to say it out loud, so she could hear it herself. You already know her answer. Nope. I tested her hormones and they were devastatingly bad. We had discovered what was causing the fire and built her hormones back to their proper levels and retested.

The next time I saw her our conversation went like this, "Doc, I'm doing so awesome, I feel amazing. I feel healthy, vital, and sexual!"

To which I replied, "Thank goodness I got rid of your menopause!"

She looked at me like I had grown a second head. I knew right away she had caught what I had said. I didn't get rid of her menopause! Menopause is a normal state of life if you live long enough. The only way for a woman to avoid it is to not reach that age in life.

It's so common for women to have a long list of symptoms of menopause: irregular periods, hot flashes, vaginal dryness, night sweats, mood changes, weight gain, thinning hair, breast fullness, they believe those symptoms are menopause. This is not menopause. This means you are sick. Your hormone levels are off. Just because the symptoms are so common, women have accepted it as normal. Don't confuse common with normal. Is PMS normal? Why then is it a "syndrome?"

When The Wellness Way doctors come along and talk about hormones and the basic biology of this transition, all of a sudden it makes sense. It doesn't matter which Wellness Way Clinic across the country you go to or which doctor you see there, we all look at it from the same perspective. The body

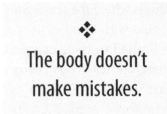

The body doesn't make mistakes.

doesn't make mistakes. If women go through those symptoms, it's a signal their bodies are struggling as they are going through the change.

Our thinking is different, and our testing approach is different. We get a complete picture of what is going on and start to find out what is throwing those hormones off so that we can help women live in that healthy, vital, sexual state of menopause. Traditional medicine can address the symptoms with synthetic hormones. Yes, the synthetic hormone works to relieve the symptoms, but the side effect is cancer. That's not a fair trade.

I'm sure some jaws will drop here, but I wish menopause for my wife. We have our four beautiful babies, and we've decided not to have anymore. I wish my wife could just go through menopause so she wouldn't have to deal with her cycle anymore. Does that sound like something any other man would wish for his wife if menopause is truly a horrible event? It is so much easier to keep a woman's hormones healthy and normal when she isn't cycling. A menopausal woman's hormone cycle isn't any different than a guy's really, it's just a flat line that's easy to keep right where it should be.

I had the blessing of helping my mom through this transition. Many people ask me what I did to help her. Well, first they ask me if I like taking care of my mom, especially through menopause. Yes! I want my mom to be healthy. I ran specific tests on her based on what I knew about her. There are multiple test options; blood, saliva, and urine. It depends on the woman and her situation. Each woman is unique and needs to be approached as such, not as a standard procedure. Based on her results there were many options to help her, and I can happily tell you her menopause experience was *normal*, not common.

The first step is changing the way you think about menopause and the way you approach your health care. If you took one of the test results I ran to a medical doctor, he'd look at the test from the perspective of which medication he is going to put you on. I appreciate that – he's trying to save you from the discomfort! What different thinking allows you to do, however, is rebuild your house, so you aren't dependent on a synthetic hormone or worse yet, a psychiatric drug for the rest of your life. You can not only survive menopause but thrive and live a life that is healthy, vital and sexual. Your body was created to go through menopause as a healthy stage of life.

The first step is changing the way you think about menopause and the way you approach your health care.

CHAPTER 13

Cholesterol is Not a Bad Guy

"My doctor says my hormones are so low I should be on these synthetic hormones," a woman tells me after a recent seminar. It's not the first time. In fact, I hear it often. So, I ask her, "Are you taking a statin or cholesterol altering medication." She said, "yes." I'm going to tell you what I told her, the several other women that came up to me that day with the same statement, and what I told the thousands of other women throughout the years: if you are taking a statin drug you can never achieve hormonal balance. Women aren't the only ones. Men are being told they need to take statins too. This is one of the biggest struggles in medicine, especially as the rate of people on statins is skyrocketing.

Over 25% of American adults over the age of forty have taken a statin drug in the past thirty days. Will statins lower your cholesterol? Yes. But let's start this conversation by first understanding cholesterol and how it got the reputation it has.

Cholesterol got a bad reputation a long time ago because it was assumed it had a role in arterial plaque formation; that idea still continues through traditional medical thinking. Cholesterol was, and still is, found in high numbers at the site of arterial plaquing. Many people thought that because it was there, it was the *cause* of the plaque formation which would eventually build up and lead to a heart attack.

We need to look deeper though, especially with all we are learning in our thinking. It's easy to blame cholesterol, but remember how the body works and that it doesn't make mistakes. We need to understand what cholesterol does, and how it works with male hormones and female hormones. This is going to be fun–something I bet you've never heard before!

Okay, we have talked about how hormones are messengers. That's what they do. Steroid hormones are a group of chemical messaging compounds produced by male and female sex organs (gonads), the adrenal glands and the kidneys (mineralocorticoid). It's your testosterone, your estrogen, your progesterone and other important hormones that keep your body functioning. We got that. Hormones are important and interconnected to your whole body. Hormones involve multiple organs. A lot of steroid hormones are produced in one organ but then go to another and are converted in that organ for function. We will learn a little more

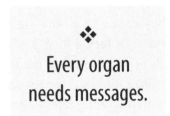

❖

Every organ needs messages.

about that later in the steroid pathway chart. It will be important to remember that every organ needs messages. There are lots of hormones bringing messages throughout your body helping it function. Steroid hormones impact a lot of your body's functions like blood pressure, bone density, and your kidneys. It's not just about male and female cycle differences.

If the message is messed up there is going to be hormonal imbalances. For example, take a hormone like estradiol. If the message delivered is too high it can develop into cancer, or too low can lead to depression or early menopause. The tissue will listen if it gets the message, but it doesn't mean it's the right message for that individual. All of our organs are controlled by messengers and the messengers can affect multiple organs. Medicine in its classification separates everything. We have heart specialists, neurologists, kidney specialists, GI specialists. We need those specialists, but the trouble we run into is they limit their scope to one organ. We need to realize messengers can affect all those organs.

You can see how important hormones are to the overall balance of the body or homeostasis. Guess where they come from. Are you ready? The building blocks of steroid hormones (and a lot of other important cells) is: cholesterol. Your body needs cholesterol, along with luteinizing hormone, to make steroid hormones. All steroid hormones are derived from cholesterol. Let's be clear—not all hormones, but all steroid hormones. Which ones are those? Sex hormones, adrenal hormones and kidney hormones. They all need cholesterol.

As you can see in the chart below, all these hormones start as cholesterol, and then become the hormones needed for a wide variety of functions. Cholesterol is a derivative. It's not bad for you. It's a building block for every steroid hormone in the body. You don't want a goal of no cholesterol. If you do, you will have depleted hormones.

STEROID HORMONE PATHWAY

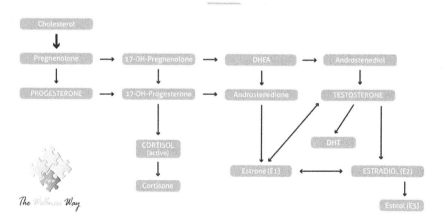

Why is my cholesterol high? That is the magic question. Your body will make cholesterol when you're under stress. It actually needs cholesterol to repair itself or when it needs more hormones. If I cut my finger and start bleeding, then my body is going to make more cholesterol to repair the wound.

When medical thinking saw the cholesterol there at the site of plaque formation, they incorrectly blamed the cholesterol. Just because the police are at the scene of a crime doesn't mean they are the ones that caused the crime. Whenever there is damage or inflammation, cholesterol has to go there to protect and heal the area. Cholesterol isn't the bad guy here, cholesterol is the police. Cholesterol is doing its job to heal and protect. The body is doing its job when it sends the cholesterol there. This misconception leads to the frequent prescription of cholesterol lowering medications. Cholesterol is needed all over and travels via the bloodstream to every single part of the body.

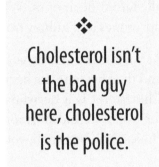

Cholesterol isn't the bad guy here, cholesterol is the police.

Let's put the pieces together. If you are a woman and your adrenals get fatigued because of stress as hormones get low, your cholesterol will go up. It's your body responding by creating what it needs to heal itself. It's not because cholesterol is this bad guy that is intruding in your body. It's not because you are eating too much cholesterol. Trust me, you can't eat enough cholesterol to make it go dangerously high. One more time—you can't eat so much cholesterol that it will go up significantly. If your cholesterol goes up, there is a physical reason why. Only 10-20% of the cholesterol in your body is associated to diet and exercise. 80+% is made by the liver. Think about it—the body does not make mistakes. Your liver makes the majority of cholesterol in your body. Do you suppose the liver would actually make something that's bad for the heart? Knowing what you now know, does that even make sense? Multiple studies have shown that dietary cholesterol does not increase coronary artery disease. Researchers are calling for guidelines to be reconsidered but unfortunately many of us are still being treated under this perspective. Cholesterol is high because the body is under stress or there is some major hormonal deficiency.

Your body makes roughly 2,000 – 3,000 milligrams of cholesterol a day. Diet change can only impact our cholesterol level by maybe 10%. Lots of you gave up eggs, shrimp and other healthy foods to have an impact on your cholesterol levels, and ultimately you were given statin drugs to lower your cholesterol—cholesterol your body needs. When I see high LDL on a guy's lab, and he has low testosterone I know what the body is doing. The body says low testosterone? What do I need to make more? Cholesterol. I will be thrilled when we all understand how this works!

The question is: what stress or hormonal deficiency is causing your body to create more cholesterol? I'm not going to drop it down with red yeast rice or statin drugs. I'm going to look into why it is high. It can be different based on the individual and very different based on gender. Anyone with chronic inflammation, stress, hormonal imbalances, autoimmune issues, leaky gut and many other health issues all NEED higher cholesterol levels to heal. The idea of creating an average or even an ideal level for cholesterol baffles me because levels can and should change dramatically when someone has some of those health issues. Cholesterol is the building block for all tissues and hormones in the body

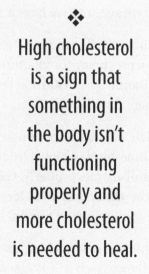

❖
High cholesterol is a sign that something in the body isn't functioning properly and more cholesterol is needed to heal.

and is not a bad thing. High cholesterol is a sign that something in the body isn't functioning properly and more cholesterol is needed to heal. Artificially lowering cholesterol with statin medication interferes with this healing process and makes people sicker.

Cholesterol has many roles beyond hormones that can be affected if we are prescribing medications to lower it. Just by looking at a few of those roles we can see how critical cholesterol is to our Swiss watch.

Cell membranes rely heavily on cholesterol. Every cell in our body is surrounded by a cell membrane. Cholesterol gives the cell membrane flexibility in addition to the strength and support necessary to maintain its shape.

We need cholesterol for optimal nerve, brain and memory function. Our nerve cells are specialized cells that transmit information throughout the body. Cholesterol allows for faster and higher quality transmission of those signals. What part of the body has the highest cholesterol? The highest amount of cholesterol is found in the brain. The brain relies on cholesterol for overall function, specifically for memory formation and retention. You can see why cholesterol becomes even more important as we age, and we have a higher demand on our brain functions.

Cholesterol is required for your body to make vitamin D. Cholesterol is a precursor for vitamin D production that is synthesized in the skin. Vitamin D is vital for your immunity along with your physical and mental well-being.

Gall bladder function is heavily reliant on the help of cholesterol. Cholesterol is converted into bile salts allowing the digestive process to emulsify fats properly. Gall bladder surgeries are on the rise! I wonder how many gall bladder surgeries could be prevented if cholesterol levels supported normal bile salt production?

This is just scratching the surface of the importance of cholesterol and why we need it. I understand this is a big shift in understanding, and some of you may still fear cholesterol. Don't govern your health care choices by fear. The drugs work on cholesterol, but the picture is so much bigger! More and more people are suffering the side effects of the drugs. It says right on the box that the side effects are low hormones, renal disease, depression, impotence and more. I see these effects

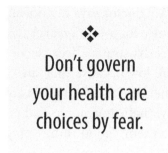

❖

Don't govern your health care choices by fear.

in patients in my office every day. I disagree that people have to live a life on these drugs, suffering the side effects. There is a different path.

Statins are shown to affect the heart. Statins interfere with the production of LDL which interfere with CoQ10. What organ does CoQ10 fuel? Your heart. Why would you take a drug for your heart that can have a bad effect on the heart? And we know it doesn't just affect the heart. Studies show that statins lower testosterone. If you lower cholesterol, you lower testosterone which increases impotence. So, statins can cause drug induced impotence. Don't worry, the drug company that makes one of the top-selling statins, Lipitor, also makes Viagra. If they make a problem, they have another drug to fix it. That's big money-making in the billions. Even though it seems like common sense, we can see in studies and anecdotal evidence that lowering cholesterol negatively impacts steroid hormones.

If a guy is taking a statin drug and his testosterone goes down, what are some of the side effects of the medication? Impotence, heart disease (the very thing it is supposed to help with), loss of motivation, weight gain. That's all on the drug packet insert. Then, we have male enhancement drugs. Let's think about that. They created the problem with one drug. Now they've created another drug to solve the problem created by the first drug. That's what they know to do, but it's not going to bring the results most people want. How many prescriptions do you need to be healthy?

"My doctor says my hormones are low because of my age." I hear that one a lot too as I travel across the country from women and men who are frustrated because of low hormones. For them, the hormones are low because they are on statins. When they get tested and follow their specific course of care, they find they can get off statin drugs and synthetic hormones and maintain hormonal balance. That's when I say to them, "good thing you got younger, your hormones are balanced!" They look at me like I'm nuts and let me know they are actually older. They are indeed—I humorously use the comment, because age doesn't have anything to do with it.

You can maintain a normal hormone balance from the day you are born until the day you die. The problem is, nobody is teaching anyone how cholesterol works, or how to keep hormones normal. Statin drugs are not just cholesterol lowering drugs, statin drugs manipulate the function of your liver's ability to make cholesterol. Cholesterol is needed to make numerous cells including steroid hormones that help your organs regulate functions like blood pressure, reproductive characteristics, metabolism, immune system, and blood sugar.

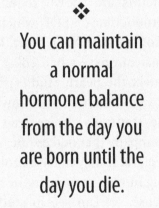

You can maintain a normal hormone balance from the day you are born until the day you die.

The use of statins has gone up, and the percentage of Americans with high cholesterol has gone down from 18.3% in 1999-2000 to 11% in 2013-2014. So why do we see rising heart disease and not lower? Cardiovascular disease is the number one cause of death in the United States for both men and women. Notice hormone concerns, depression and blood pressure are also going up. One in four Americans are taking statins and they want to increase that number. You can see the results now that we realize cholesterol isn't the bad guy.

If you are taking a statin drug, you may have lower cholesterol, but you can never achieve hormonal balance. This is just one part of the body, but as we know the Swiss watch principle means every part plays a role that can impact all the other parts. Stopping just one gear has a tremendous impact on the entire body.

CHAPTER 14

The Liver is a Machine

Do you remember that movie, *The Horse Whisperer?* The one where the guy could figure out what was going on without them being able to say it? Well, one day, I had two different follow-up appointments with two different women. They each said to me, "You are like my own Hormone Whisperer." After that I started to see it posted in comments online. I didn't ask to be called that. It's not that I don't like the nickname. It's kind of cool, but I worry people miss the point. You have made it far enough into the book to know that I don't treat hormones. I disagree with the whole idea of looking at just the symptoms and treating those. I look at the whole body to find out what is happening with everything, including the hormones.

It's a Swiss watch. There are many organs that impact every piece of our overall health. What's the secret that made me The Hormone Whisperer? The liver.

The liver is a machine and is very important for the bigger picture. The liver performs over 500 vital functions for the body. The liver does way more than what people give it credit for. Most people just think of it as a detoxing organ, which is true. It clears

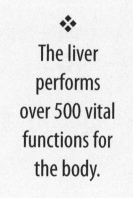

❖

The liver performs over 500 vital functions for the body.

out harmful toxins, like alcohol and medications from the blood. Every day our bodies are bombarded with all kinds of toxins in our food, clothing, body products, environment, and workplace that can overload our liver. It works hard for detoxing but there is so much more! It produces blood clotting factors and is needed for cholesterol production. The liver stores energy, vitamins, enzymes, and minerals like iron. Did you know the liver is important for hormone conversion? It's a converting machine!

There is all this crazy stuff that happens in the liver to make up all those hormones that make up so much of who we are. They don't just show up for work, they are created by your amazing body. So, we know that cholesterol is essential for steroid hormone production. We also know cholesterol is made in the liver, which is part one why the liver is important for healthy hormones, but it doesn't end there. After being produced in the liver, the cholesterol is excreted into the blood. That cholesterol goes off to the adrenal glands and is made into pregnenolone. Pregnenolone is known as the mother hormone. Why is it the *mother hormone*? Let's bring back that chart from the cholesterol chapter.

STEROID HORMONE PATHWAY

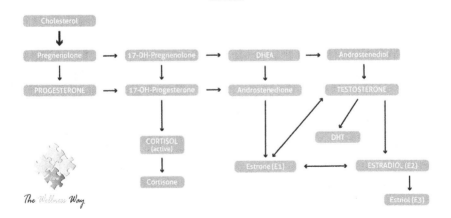

See pregnenolone is the next step on that chart and pregnenolone has the opportunity to become all these different hormones. It is the precursor to estrogens, testosterone, progesterone, cortisol and all the other steroid hormones. How does that happen? Once pregnenolone is produced, it goes into the bloodstream. Some of it goes to the nervous system where it is used to make myelin sheath. The main job of the myelin sheath is to protect the important stuff like your brain. If we lower cholesterol, we lower your pregnenolone which could leave your brain unprotected. The rest of your pregnenolone eventually makes its way to the testicles or adrenals

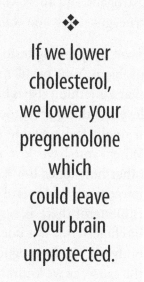

❖

If we lower cholesterol, we lower your pregnenolone which could leave your brain unprotected.

where it is converted into testosterone, and to the liver where it is converted into other steroid hormones. What is happening in the body and the liver can have an impact on what those hormones become.

Here's a real-life example for guys that will clarify the importance of what's happening in the liver. If you have lots of testosterone production from your testicles and your adrenals, that doesn't necessarily mean your testosterone levels will be great. That testosterone eventually makes its way to the liver. The function and nutrients there can impact how it is converted there. If you have an enzyme called 5 alpha-reductase enzyme you will convert that testosterone to DHT too quickly. Too much DHT has been linked to baldness, acne, and other problems. That's not all that can go wrong once testosterone makes its way to the liver. The number one thing that accelerates the conversion of testosterone to estrogen is an enzyme called aromatase which is increased by insulin. What causes increased insulin? We talked about this earlier. It's sugar. If guys produce too much of that enzyme, they will convert that testosterone they have been working hard for into estrogens and they will end up with a chest like a woman's. Sad but true, guys! Yes, you want to be sure your liver is functioning optimally.

That's why taking testosterone supplements doesn't address the actual problem. Your problem wasn't that you were short on testosterone, it's that something else is happening and that is affecting your testosterone levels. Taking a synthetic hormone doesn't get you back to normal. It might feel amazing at first, but it doesn't get you back to normal. When you have low pregnenolone, it's very common to have the other hormones low too. That's why you never want to synthetically lower your cholesterol. Like we have talked about, if you have excess cholesterol there is a stress in the body that has led to that increase in cholesterol. If a doctor synthetically lowers your cholesterol, your body can't make pregnenolone. When I see high cholesterol, I look for the cause; as we know that can often be mental stress. Here's that chart that looks at hormone conversion.

STEROID HORMONE PATHWAY

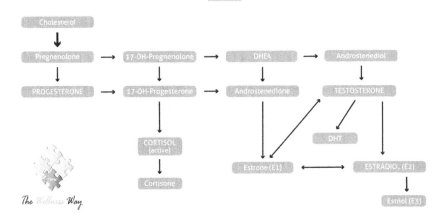

Look at that middle row where pregnenolone can either take the pathway to convert into your estrogens or it can convert into cortisol. Remember, cortisol is your stress hormone. This kicks in when you need it. Say your house is on fire. Your cholesterol is going to skyrocket to make pregnenolone and your body is going to go into fight or flight mode. It's supposed to for you to be able to survive. Your cortisol and adrenaline are going to kick in to get you out of that house. That pregnenolone is going down the pathway to make those stress hormones. It's how your body was designed to survive.

Who has the most mental stress? Ladies! Chronic mental stress leaves us in that fight or flight mode. The body doesn't know the difference between whether it is a fire causing that stress or if it's because of all the everyday stresses life throws at you. It just knows stress. So, a lot of mental stress will cause the pregnenolone to be stolen for the production of your stress hormones.

This pathway is why a man can give up soda and lose twenty pounds in a week and a woman can give up soda and nothing happens. Sugar is a major stressor for men, but it's not her major stressor. That's why it doesn't matter if a woman eats good or eats poorly, she can still gain weight. Your adrenals can steal pregnenolone and stress can drain your hormones.

We can't talk about each hormone and every enzyme that affects every hormone pathway. A lot happens in the liver. What is important to know is that a lot can be happening in the liver that can show us why those hormone levels are off. Let's look at estrogen dominance specifically related to progesterone. What causes estrogen dominance? It could be phytoestrogens like soy, plastics, toxicity, a liver pathway

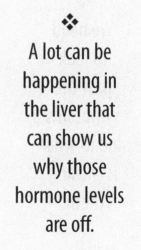

❖

A lot can be happening in the liver that can show us why those hormone levels are off.

issue where liver doesn't break them down and it could be too much sugar. These all are affecting conversion change but what are they ultimately affecting? They are affecting the liver. They are affecting the liver's ability to process and regulate and normalize what the levels should be at in an optimal scenario. Our lifestyle and the 3-T's ultimately affect the liver; that reflects in the hormones.

If you want to have great hormones, it's essential to have great liver function. I can't give you a magic herb that will fix your hormones. Your medical doctor can give you a drug that will change your hormones, but that's not a true magical fix either. A lot of hormone issues are revealed in the function of the liver. The thing is, your liver isn't kept in a bubble. Yes, if you have a bad liver you can have bad hormones, but there is more. The gallbladder is essential for liver function. It stores the bile that breaks down the toxins from the liver. If you have a bad gallbladder, or no gallbladder, you can have bad hormones. The stomach is needed to help flush out the toxins so that the liver can function properly. If you have a bad stomach, you can have bad hormones.

❖

We need to look past the symptoms and to what is causing them.

How did I become The Hormone Whisperer? I didn't worry about hormones. I worried about all the things that affect your hormones. As you can see by just looking at a small part of what the liver does, it plays a major role in the hormones and the body's function overall. Just like the rest of your organ systems that make up your unique Swiss watch. We need to look past the symptoms and to what is causing them. It's sad that most readers won't find out all of this until they are already sick. Anything you do to reduce irritation or inflammation will put a lesser demand on the hormonal system.

CHAPTER 15

Detoxing in a Toxic World

We live in a toxic world. Some people say it's really not that toxic, and some people say our bodies can handle the toxicity. I disagree with both groups. They've introduced over 80,000 hazardous toxins since the industrial revolution. 4.5 billion pounds of pesticides are sprayed on crops every year. We just talked about how the liver has hundreds of jobs and one of those roles is a part of the detox process. Since the body is like a Swiss watch, those toxins aren't just impacting the liver; they are affecting the whole body. Everything works together. If you have a problem in one system, it is going to impact others. If you have a problem with the digestive system, that's going to impact your other gears. Your body can't function properly if there are a lot of toxins. Juice cleanses are popular, but they aren't an actual detox. If you haven't done a proper detox overseen by a professional, then you probably have a high toxic load.

Every choice we make is either adding to our toxic load or supporting our body. The majority of my patients aren't functioning anywhere near 100% and a lot of that starts with their toxic load. How did toxins get in your body? We are exposed to toxins daily and can acquire them from our environment by breathing, ingesting, or coming into physical contact with them. Also, most drugs, food additives, and allergens can create toxic elements in the body.

When a new patient comes into my office, they have already encountered numerous toxins adding to their very heavy toxic load. So, when I tell them they have to give up Mountain Dew it might be painful for them, but it is just the tip of their toxic iceberg.

When their eyes flutter open after hitting snooze for the third time, their nose is breathing toxins from the laundry soap and dryer sheet residue on their pillow case. They stumble to the bathroom to brush their teeth with toothpaste that has fluoride, which is a known neurotoxin. Then they hop in the shower. Their shower curtain is likely made with phthalates that they will breathe in. They squirt some chemical-laden body wash in their hands and slather it on. Then they lather up their hair with shampoos that can have one of over 10,000 chemicals that are commonly used in personal care products. How many more products will they use before they leave the bathroom? That varies but the average woman uses twelve per day, which means she's potentially been exposed to hundreds of toxins before she left the bathroom.

Then it is time for breakfast. The average American diet does not include a breakfast of whole, organic foods. It's usually a prepackaged meal and processed cereals. Nobody tells people the impact the ingredients in processed foods has on them. If you are eating three times a day, there's three more times you're opening yourself to toxins. If you aren't eating organic, whole foods then you are eating a lot of pesticides and chemicals.

What kinds of pesticides and chemicals?

- Did you know DDT is still used in Asia, South America and Africa—sure, we don't use it in the U.S., but do we get food from other places? We sure do!

- Glyphosate is the #1 pesticide used in America and more commonly known as Round-up. With the surge of GMOs that are resistant to pesticides your breakfast comes with an extra serving of Round-up.

- Atrazine # 2 pesticide is used in America with 26 million pounds used on U.S. crops each year.

- Artificial colors and flavors are common in our foods. When the public becomes informed of specifics that may be harmful, they just change the name to make it more difficult to find.

- MSG is not just in Chinese food. It's in lots of processed foods and is an excitotoxin that has been linked to brain diseases like Alzheimer's, Lou Gehrig's disease, Parkinson's disease and learning disabilities

- Red dye #40 triggers hyperactivity in children

- Blue dye #2 has been linked to brain tumors.

Next in my patient's day: how many pollutants did they breathe in on the drive to my office? Too many. I know, I hear it coming... "But Doc, didn't you say the body was built to detox naturally?" I did and that's still true. Here's the thing, our bodies can only handle so much before it becomes difficult for the body to naturally detoxify. Everybody has a bucket and once your bucket is full it gets harder to detoxify. What's your bucket? Let me explain.

There's a theory that explains this need for detoxification called "The Bucket Theory." Picture for a moment that every person has a "toxin bucket" that they are born with. At birth, some people have buckets that are somewhat empty, some are about half-full, and others are nearly full. Why are some people's toxin buckets nearly full at birth? Heavy metals and other toxins can pass

When a baby is born the umbilical cord will contain an average of 280 toxins.

through the placenta to the baby. When a baby is born the umbilical cord will contain an average of 280 toxins.

Metal fillings, metals from vaccines and prescription drugs, cadmium from smoking or just being around cigarette smoke, lead paint, and aluminum from soda pop are all examples of toxins that mom could have passed to you through her placenta. If your bucket is half or nearly full at birth, would you agree with me that it would not take many more toxins to fill it up, and cause it to start overflowing? This is why we are seeing so many more sick children today! When the bucket "splashes over" you will see outward manifestations of toxic overload occurring in the body.

Potential Signs of Toxic Overload:

- Asthma and seasonal allergies
- Cognitive problems
- Depression
- Anxiety
- Fatigue
- Headaches
- Memory problems
- Chronic pain
- Autoimmune disease
- Weight fluctuations
- Eczema
- Infertility
- Cancer
- Chemical sensitivity
- Chronic infection

- Diabetes
- Fibromyalgia
- Skin reactions
- Food allergies
- High blood pressure
- Hormonal imbalances

We talked about how a person can start out their day encountering 100's of toxins. If these aren't detoxed, they build up in the body. These built-up toxins can lead to many different health conditions. Even if you were born with a nearly empty bucket, with all the toxins surrounding us, it's only a matter of time before your bucket will fill up. Don't wait until your bucket overflows!

CHRISTY'S THOUGHTS

When I got pregnant, I was still in the process of changing my diet, household and body care products, and environment around me. What I didn't realize at that time was how toxic I was from my past exposure to lead paint/pipes, aluminum, and other heavy metals, as well as having a messed up immune system due to past antibiotics, and a diet that included foods that were either toxic (full of chemicals and pesticides) or toxic to me due to food allergies I didn't know I had. So, I passed toxins and an unhealthy immune system to my child. Did I have mommy guilt? Perhaps, but let me explain something that might help other mothers experiencing a similar circumstance. The fact that you are reading this book right now means that you realize that changes need to happen.

At the time that our oldest was born, we were already on a path towards homeostasis, and I knew that I was given a gift: a child. Despite all of my past health challenges. And with that gift, I was given a responsibility to continue to learn and grow in order to make sure our children would grow up healthier than me. When each of our children were born, I knew they had some toxins in their buckets. As a result, we purposefully chose to limit their toxin exposures in all areas of our lives and build their immune systems naturally. Don't look back with guilt once you learn truth. Instead be grateful you are learning it now and make changes moving forward. Raise your children with that 'toxin bucket' image in mind and teach them how to reduce their exposure to toxins as they are growing up so that when they are ready to have children, they won't be passing on a half or nearly full bucket of toxins to your grandchildren. If this is the first time you've heard anything about toxicity, I pray that you take this new knowledge to heart and share it with your loved ones to create a healthier future for generations to come

If you take the time to assist your body in detoxification, you will help in emptying out your bucket, which will reduce the toxic stress on your body and allow it to function better. Once function is restored, your body will again be able to naturally detox itself, to some extent, on a regular basis. Now that doesn't mean after a detox that you can go back to eating non-organic, heavily processed foods or other toxic bad habits.

Built-up hormones from a stressed-out liver can be stressors on the body.

When you make a commitment to your health, it's a lifelong commitment. Every day your body is working to get rid of both external toxins and internal toxins. Yes, internal! Did that surprise you? Toxins can come from within. Built-up hormones from a stressed-out liver can be stressors on the body. Our overall health is a reflection of the health of our cells and their ability to work together in harmony to maintain balance.

Our cells constantly take in nutrients and oxygen from the blood to work, grow, or create products, and that process gives off wastes. In addition to the wastes that normal function produces, we are further burdened by toxins absorbed from the intestinal tract. Poor food choices, poor digestion, and dysbiosis (parasitic, bacterial, and fungal infections) can make a mess of the intestine which makes it harder to detox. Together these absorbed toxins and the wastes produced by cells are discharged from the bloodstream into the surrounding tissues, "the cellular garbage dump," where they sit until they are transported to the organs of elimination for final disposal.

You see why minimizing your toxic exposure and making sure your body is detoxing properly is so important. It's not a given, and it could very well be the reason you are sick. Or maybe you don't think you are sick. It's just old age, right? I can't tell you how many times I have had patients go through the detox, and not only did the symptoms for the health problem they came in for alleviate, but they tell me they feel years younger. Sometimes twenty, thirty or even forty years younger! That's another happy side effect of being healthy. They often lose weight too. Toxins can cause weight gain. Toxins get into fatty tissue. The body holds on to these toxins as a defense mechanism, so they aren't released into the bloodstream. Once you get the toxins out of your system, your body won't hold on to that fat anymore. That's long-term health benefits, not just water weight loss!

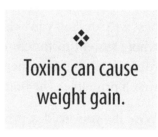

Toxins can cause weight gain.

These are benefits you can't get from a cleanse. You wouldn't believe how many times I hear from people who have done a cleanse. You might lose some bloating, and may even get back a bit of energy, but you can't get a good detox from a cleanse. You may be surprised to hear you could actually end up making yourself even sicker. There is a lot of confusion out there with all the fad cleanses. Let's take a look at the difference between a cleanse and a detox. I have another analogy to help you to better understand!

Picture a long hallway lined with doors... now picture Mr. Janitor sweeping and scrubbing that hallway. This is what a cleanse does–it simply cleans the hallway. Now picture that same hallway lined with doors. This time Mr. Janitor not only sweeps and scrubs the hallway, but he also opens the doors and sweeps/scrubs the rooms that line the hallway. This is what a detox does. A cleanse may not require doctor supervision, but they may inadvertently harm delicate systems. The GI tract is a delicate ecosystem comprised of many kinds of bacteria. When people innocently use a cleanse to clean out their colon for example, they don't realize that they may be clearing out some good bacteria, altering the delicate ecosystem and ultimately making themselves even more sick. And the janitor didn't even do a good job cleaning!

When doing a real detox, we are focusing on all the detox pathways and all the organs. We are going to help clean up the whole body the best we can. You can't clean just one room or hall way and expect the whole system to function better. Eventually the mess from the other rooms spills out into the room you cleaned. Keep thinking of the Swiss watch principle! The body works as a whole.

Why do you need a professional to oversee your detox? While it is good to minimize your exposure to toxins by upgrading your diet to organic, whole foods and using cleaner personal care products, you can't just dive into a detox. You have a lifetime of filling and probably overflowing that bucket; there may be some damage that needs to be addressed before you go pushing toxins around.

A proficient doctor will assess and test your body to find out if it is ready for a detox. You need to know if your body is functioning well enough to handle the detox and has the nutrients to properly do so.

We check for food allergies that lead to inflammation and leaky gut. The most common area we have to improve is the GI. If you are like most people, you may have gut issues. Many people have bloating, gas, diarrhea, constipation and other signs of gut issues. What's an easy way to know if you have gut issues? Take a look at your poop. Are you pooping at least two or three times a day? Does it look like chocolate soft serve ice cream? If it doesn't, you are not ready for a detox.

Doing that detox before your gut is ready is a very bad idea. During those first days you're drawing toxins that may be stuck in the fat tissues or other organs when you force a detox. If you try to pull those out too soon, without your GI being properly healed, all that stuff can actually leak back in the system and make you really sick.

CHRISTY'S THOUGHTS

Not so funny story about a friend who insisted that she wanted to do a detox, but to save money, she decided to go to a local health food store and buy a cheap one instead of doing the one through our office where she would be monitored by one of our doctors. She ended up in the emergency room in intense pain and became very sick as a result. The cheap 'detox' wiped out all her beneficial bacteria and caused infections that didn't exist prior to the unsupervised 'detox'. She may have saved some cash up front, but was it worth it?

I also know someone who constantly does cleanses. At one point her health had deteriorated so bad that she also ended up in the emergency room. She continued to insist that the cleanses were helping...I disagree. Moral of the stories? Your body is an intricate ecosystem of bacteria, organs and systems that work together to create homeostasis. If something messes with the complex ecosystem, the body will try to bring itself back to homeostasis. If you are feeling 'off', don't try to guess at what will fix what's going on in your body...you need to be properly tested so you don't inadvertently make it worse.

The gut is a very important part of your body's detox assembly line. Yes! Think of it like an assembly line. It's not just as simple as drinking some juice and flushing the toxins out. There's important work happening there. It's a multi-system job with three phases. A detox covers the whole body. All your organs, your blood circulation and your lymphatic system takes the detox to every corner of your body. There are some key players to support.

Key Detox Players:

It's not just as simple as drinking some juice and flushing the toxins out. There's important work happening there.

- Liver– the main filter or cleaner
- Lungs – processing O2 and H2O
- Gallbladder – creates bile
- Kidneys – needed for blood filtration
- Intestines – microbiome has to be functioning to push the toxins out
- Blood vessels and lymphatic tissue

All of these have to be functioning for a detox to be effective. What happens during a detox? Here are the basics:

Phase one is what we call the *biotransformation phase*. It's the phase where the body breaks things down from fat-soluble toxins. Here's another analogy for you. You just made some really tasty bacon for breakfast. Sizzled to perfection. Instead of cleaning the pan right away, you sat down and ate that bacon. I mean if you don't eat it right away, someone else will. When you go back to clean the pan, it's crusty grease. You can't just spray water on it. You need dish soap to break it down. That's what your body does in this phase. It breaks down those fat-soluble toxins. That's why phase two is important.

Phase two is what we call the *conjugation phase.* This is the building things up phase. After phase one, your body is left with a bunch of broken-down metabolites that can be more toxic than the original fat-soluble toxins you started with. There are a bunch of metabolic pathways that make sure those broken-down toxins bind to natural enzymes or substances created by your liver. Some bodies are better at that than others. If your liver has been stressed for years it can take a toll on this process. Your liver and body need support during this process to make sure those metabolites from phase one are bound so they make it to the exit. If they aren't, then they are recirculated into the body. That will make you feel very crappy.

Getting shown the door, or the excretion process, is the last important step in this process. You see this step happen every day in the way of stool, urine and sweat. Smaller toxins that travel in the blood go to the kidneys to be filtered. Larger molecules are excreted through bile that comes from the gall bladder into the small intestine. If we are pushing toxins into intestines, we need something to push them through the back door. Vegetables, beans and lots of other fibrous foods are really important during the detox. We don't tell you to eat veggies because we want you to be miserable. I don't get excited about veggies, but our body

When you put the hard work into making sure your body is functioning, you think more about what you are exposing it to.

needs them. I can't say this enough, if you don't get the toxins out, they can make you sick.

Can you see how critical each part of the detox process is and why it is important to support the body through each step? I bet you also see why minimizing your exposure to toxins is so important. When you put the hard work into making sure your body is functioning, you think more about what you are exposing it to. The body should be functioning at 100% and it can't do that if it's not effectively detoxing.

CHAPTER 16

Say It... I Disagree

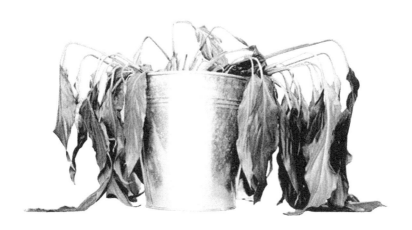

What do you think this plant needs? Water. Why didn't you say drugs or surgery? Why didn't you say horse hormones? Most people understand more about how to take care of a plant than their own body. That's frustrating for me. Traditional doctors do their best to manage symptoms and minimize pain. It's honestly amazing what they can do, but what they're never taught to do is support the body to bring it back to normal. It's not how they are trained to look at or approach a health condition. They are trained to go in with their ax and hose to do what they were taught to do, to save your life. That's ok! When your body is on fire, you'll be grateful for that axe and hose—I know I was grateful they could help my wife with her pain, until we could get her back to normal. Both sides of this conversation are important—stopping the fire, and rebuilding the house. I disagree with simply putting out the fire.

Every day, couples are told they will not be able to have a baby. Then there are the patients who hear they need to be on a drug for their high cholesterol. Girls are told birth control is the answer to their period problems. People are told they are fat because of genetics. Divorce rates are going higher because society tells us men and women are the same. Menopause is a change that is feared. Men are told testosterone goes down as they age. Women are told there is nothing wrong with them even though they have a laundry list of symptoms. I disagree with all of this and so much more. Don't you?

Don't you agree that there needs to be another approach? One that builds the body? I want this approach to be known all over. Everyone deserves it! You deserve individual care that treats you, not just the average person. Your body is a Swiss watch with different gears and a unique makeup; that means an individual set of hormones. It means individual triggers and individual circumstances. Now that you know of a different way to look at the body you have powerful information that can change the future of your health.

> ❖
> **You deserve individual care that treats you, not just the average person.**

Patty's Story

After 11 years of infertility, exploratory surgeries and rounds of IVF, I was feeling done. It was hard wanting to be pregnant, seeing pregnant strangers or being with a friend who was expecting a baby. I had been told by the IVF doctors I'd never be able to carry a baby in my womb. They told me I would have to look into a surrogate or adopt. I wanted to have a hysterectomy. If I couldn't use my female organs, I didn't want them.

When we had found The Wellness Way and Dr. Patrick, a cancelation enabled us to get in right away. I knew it was meant to be!

We learned a whole new lifestyle at The Wellness Way. The approach was completely different. From all that we learned, I have referred my sister, a neighbor, people with cancer and those with other health challenges. While some people are opposed to trying anything different, others have great results with The Wellness Way.

We had several people who were skeptical and told us it wouldn't work. I faced my own challenge. I worked in the dairy industry. Due to my allergies, I had to eliminate dairy from my diet. I often heard "don't bite the hand that feeds you;" but I had to do what was right for my body.

We are now expecting our second baby and weren't even trying – it just happened. We weren't trying but we also weren't not trying. We figured since it took 11 years to have our son, he would be our only child. Then I started waking up with nausea and wasn't feeling well. I was 8 weeks along before I realized I was pregnant.

When I share my Wellness Way story, a lot of people are concerned about insurance coverage. I tell them all it's worth it. If this is what you want, and this is your dream in life, then there really is no dollar amount. When we went through IVF, we spent tens of thousands of dollars. All the medications were out of pocket as well. When I talked to my insurance company about the IVF, I was told having a child isn't a necessity of life and they wouldn't cover it. Now, I tell people to put that money toward fixing your body the right way. Let it work the way it should and treat it right. You only have one body.

*At time of publishing, Patty was pregnant with baby number three!

Hope Restored

I want to share more of Patty's story with you. As she and her husband Josh tried to start their family, they faced some heartache. Eleven years ago, Patty and her husband Josh tried to get pregnant. After trying for eleven years, guess what happened, nothing. She went to the medical doctors. They only have two tools. They gave her medications, did she get pregnant? No. She didn't. So, they only had one tool left, they decided to do IVF therapy. They extracted three eggs from her ovaries and fertilized them, then they implanted one. Any guess how much that cost? $20,000. Insurance covers nothing.

Patty paid the $20,000 and it did not work. They implanted the second egg for $20,000 and that didn't work. The doctors told Patty and her husband that they had one more egg left, and they felt bad for her since she had already spent $40,000, so they'd do the last one for $5,000. But before they did this, the doctors said they'd heard about this guy in Green Bay, Wisconsin. They were talking about me! They didn't really know what I do, but they told her, "He gets crazy results."

Patty and her husband came into The Wellness Way. As we were going through her medical records, I asked her some very basic questions. "Did they test your hormones?"

"No."

Well, they actually had tested one of them, but it was incomplete testing. We tested all her hormones and found the imbalance. I started the process of finding the triggers and what she needed to do to balance her hormones. It took time to rebuild her body. After nine months we retested her. She was regaining healthy levels of hormones; I sent her back to her doctor. They did the last in-vitro and she got pregnant. I was so happy for her and Josh!

Here's what followed. Medicine has standards they do with everyone. One of the standards they do with IVF is to give the woman hormone shots to keep her pregnant. Why? They have to force the body to keep the pregnancy. This is a standard because, unless the mother is working with a doctor like those in our Wellness Way network, the body hasn't been brought to a place of healthy function. Standard medicine is trying to help, and make sure they manipulate those hormone levels to maintain the pregnancy. Josh, Patty's husband, called me and was concerned they wanted to do these hormone shots. "Doc, is this okay?" I told him, "Her labs are normal; the shots now will make her abnormal again, and she'll get sick. "

She went back to the doctor, shared her concerns, and the doctor told her "Dr. Patrick is hurting you, don't go back to him. You have to do this. If you do not, we won't take care of you." You know what? He was trying to make sure she did what he knew, based on his experience.

See guys they don't see the body like we do, so they don't understand this approach. They haven't been trained to and some might even stop you from asking questions. A doctor who doesn't allow you to question his approach is wrong. What have those other doctors done? They've tried, but their thinking is focused on the fire. We rebuild the body and support the

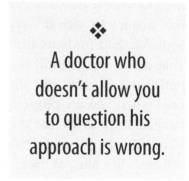

❖

A doctor who doesn't allow you to question his approach is wrong.

body's natural ability to heal. This leads to places traditional medicine is unfamiliar with.

So, what happened with Patty? She was scared so she listened to them and got the shots. Six weeks later, in October, that baby died. My heart broke for her. The doctor conclusively told her, "You can't have children," and left. He had nothing left to offer her. Imagine how she felt in that moment. She had trusted this doctor, and he had no answers for her.

She went into a deep depression after she lost the baby. Josh texted me and called me often saying, "I can't get Patty out of bed she's so depressed." I told him to leave her be, she had to get her stress down. It was a normal reaction both physically and mentally to what she had just been through. She lost a baby and the idea of a family—she was going through tremendous physical stress. A month later I hadn't heard from them. Then Josh reached out to me again. "Doc, Patty's finally getting up and around. You made the most sense to us even when the other doctors didn't understand your thinking. My wife was the happiest and healthiest when she was with you. I understand we can't have a baby, but I'd rather have my wife happy and healthy than sick with no child."

I told him, "I know what the doctors said, but I disagree. Don't tell your wife that though. She doesn't need to hear that right now. We need to remove the stressors and get her body functioning." Her body was struggling with the synthetic hormones she had been injected with. We had to detox her and build her hormones back properly. That detox was painful for her; there was a lot that needed to be pulled out. She felt like she was going to die. A detox can be very hard when you are properly pulling all of the toxins. February 8th, I called Patty so we could redo her labs. She said that she and Josh were going to go on vacation to Mexico for three weeks. I told her to call me when she got back.

March came around and all of a sudden, I got a text message from Patty. She said, "Dr. Patrick, I was at work today and my boobs were sore, I was tired, and I got nauseous, so I went to Walgreens and I bought seven pregnancy tests and they are all positive. How did that happen?!" I told her she was a little old for the talk about the birds and the bees and she should know how it happened! I laugh every time I tell that part of the story!

Recently she sent me a picture of her son, "Joshua wanted to say hi to his favorite doctor!"

Why am I his favorite doctor? Because their story had a happy ending for them, but their story was far from easy. The other doctors had given up hope and offered his parents no hope of having children. Their thinking and philosophy were different than the one Patty and her husband needed. They are very good at their jobs, but does their thinking get you where you truly want to be? Back to normal function and health?

There is no other approach? I disagree! I'm so saddened by people being sick, infertile, unhappy, and divorced. I want to live in a world where rates of cancer, heart disease and all common, chronic diseases are actually *decreasing*. We have to change the direction that we are going in and it has to start somewhere. Even if that just means saying, I disagree.

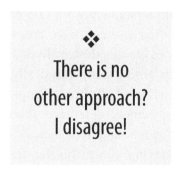

Take Comfort

People are uncomfortable with the concept of disagreement. It has negative connotations, and even just the thought can bring on feelings of anxiety, anger, stress, and tension. However, disagreement does not have to be a bad thing – in fact, when done respectfully, it's actually a very good thing! Why do I say that? Because the ability to disagree and walk through constructive conflict is a gift – it means you have a choice. It means we have the opportunity to learn and grow, and pursue new things. Things that may be different than the norm, but hold promise. Imagine, knowing what you know now after going through this book, and not having the option to disagree. Imagine being told nothing can be done, and the door is shut forever. Imagine a doctor looking at you and your very real symptoms, telling you it's all in your head, and it's the end. Imagine being handed a laundry list of prescriptions with side-effects worse than the actual illness, and being told it doesn't matter, you'll be fine, and there's simply no other options. Maybe that hopeless scene has already been a part of your story – it surely has been for tens of thousands of other people, and is one of the reasons I am so passionate about this topic. This, right here, right now. This is the part of the story where we get to make a change.

Health is a very emotional topic, and understandably so. It's extremely personal and can have consequences that can literally destroy lives; be it financially, emotionally, physically, or a combination of all three. People can become extremely defensive about health decisions, and rely heavily on emotions. Having come this far in your understanding, however, let me ask you a question: do you think the traditional medical way of thinking has been bringing us closer to health? Emotional as it may be, looking at the statistics, there is no question: the fire department is excellent, but we are sorely lacking in carpenters. Our emergency care is second to none, but if we are increasingly dying from long-term, chronic conditions, something is still wrong. We are not healthy.

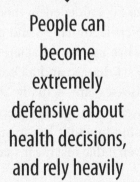

People can become extremely defensive about health decisions, and rely heavily on emotions.

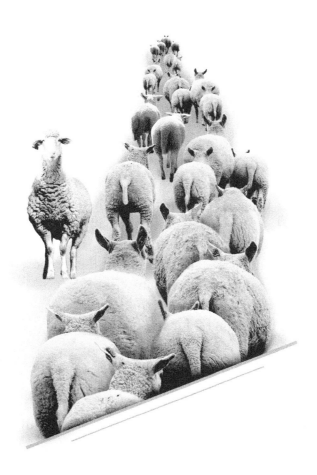

Taking the conventional path is easy. If you don't count the frustration, heartache, and hit-and-miss results, you will find it a comforting path. You will be like the vast majority of the herd, and people are very comfortable with being in the herd. Everyone going one way, traveling together with little resistance along the clearly marked path. Here's the problem though – where's the herd going? Are they taking you where you **really** want to go? Now that you've made it to the end of this book, I hope you realize just how important those questions are.

In the picture above, there's a sheep thinking differently. He has his head raised high, and clearly has ideas that differ from the herd. While the other sheep are being blindly led, that single sheep is changing his story. This is how I picture life. So many people are blindly following a path, in the pursuit of health. The path is a series of misinformation, bad habits, poor health advice, and however well-intended, the intent doesn't matter because the actual results are disastrous. It's a bleak picture, but that's what makes this exciting – the story isn't over.

In the picture above, I think you know which sheep I identify with – the one thinking differently! I hope by now I have provided enough evidence and provoked enough thought that you are thinking differently too. Unlike the image though, there is more than just one who is bold. There are many of us. Actually, there are hundreds of thousands of us – across the country, and across the globe, all thinking differently and taking a stand. Realizing there's more to be done, realizing there are different, better answers, and getting incredible results as we go. This is where the story changes, for the better! Not just my story, your story. Your story is so important! Not just to you, but to everyone around you. Your story reaches your loved ones and community, and has the power to change lives. This is where we impact not only our generation, but generations to come. Now, more than ever, it's time to take a stand, think differently, and say I disagree!

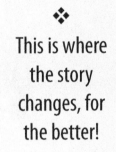

This is where the story changes, for the better!

Nicole's Story

So many things are clear when looking back. Hindsight is definitely 20/20. Since puberty, I have struggled with my periods. In high school they were regular in terms of time, but they were also painful leading to missed school. I also struggled with anemia so severe I was seeing specialists, and having colonoscopies to find the source of low iron levels. These specialists never found the cause of the anemia and why I would frequently pass out. I now understand my periods were way too heavy and I was losing too much blood.

My mom approved the use of birth control to help steady my period. I did find some relief for the couple of years that I was on it. I left for college and started planning a wedding. I knew that my periods were inconsistent. I wanted to have a more regular life and let my body adjust, find a normal rhythm. I knew this would take some time so 6 months before my husband and I got married, I went off birth control.

After stopping the birth control, I went months without getting a period. I was a virgin at the time, but I was convinced I had somehow gotten pregnant. When it did come it was incredibly painful and it would then be months before having another one.

I finally went to see a Nurse Practitioner about the issues. She did some further testing and I was diagnosed with Polycystic Ovary Syndrome (PCOS). Because I had such irregular periods, they told me it would likely be very difficult for me to conceive. This news was devastating. I found out a few months before I was supposed to get married. I had the conversation with my fiancé. I knew he had always wanted to have children.

"I don't know if I'm going to be able to have kids. Are you sure you still want to marry me even if this is something I can't give you?" I asked him. He was surprised but said whatever it takes, we'll figure this out together. When I was younger and had gone on mission trips, one thing they asked us during team building exercises was our biggest fear. My biggest fear was always that I wouldn't be able to have kids. When we were going through pre-marital counseling, I said I didn't want kids. I think it was a defense mechanism. I believed that if I didn't want children, it wouldn't be painful to find out that I couldn't. Through that pre-marital counseling, I realized that I really did want kids. The reality that I might be unable to have children felt like a nightmare.

We started our marriage in this stage of not knowing what our future family would look like. During that first year of marriage while dealing with the diagnosis of PCOS, I gained 70 pounds. When we had been married two years, I was still in college, so we weren't actively trying to have a baby. Because I knew that the possibility existed that it would be difficult for me to conceive, we decided we weren't going to prevent any pregnancy with birth control. We decided that if it happens, it happens. A baby would be God's gift to us. Reality was, all these people around me were getting pregnant that didn't want to get pregnant. I was having a hard time processing our situation. We were married. We had a good home for welcoming babies. Why wasn't this happening for us? I went into a depression thinking parenthood was never going to happen for us. One night I was just lying in bed and I started praying. "God, I do feel like I'm going to have a baby someday, but could you give me a dream or a sign or something to get my mind in the right mindset if adoption is my future? Please bring me some sort of clarity. I'm afraid of the unknown." That night I dreamed I was in a dark room with my eyes closed, rubbing my belly and feeling that distinct kick of a baby growing in the womb. I felt in my dream that someone had said, "His name is Simon." I woke up wondering what it meant. Simon is very specific and a name I wouldn't normally have picked for a baby. However, God has named a lot of people throughout history. I looked up the meaning of the name Simon; He has heard. I was stunned. The next month I found out I was pregnant with my son. Of course, we named him Simon!

After Simon was born, I was still very overweight. My doctor prescribed Metformin, a prescription often given to people who have PCOS. It helps insulin resistance, a common concern with PCOS. It gave me digestive upset. I never knew when I would have diarrhea and it was awful. After a month, I stopped taking the Metformin and decided I was going to have to live with the situation and deal with it. I felt like at this time, God was whispering to me, "get your body back to healthy and the second one will come." I tried everything. Exercising. Drinking meal replacement shakes. Eating healthy. I was doing all I knew to do. You know the standard to get your body healthy—diet and exercise. I lost 20 pounds on my own, but it was difficult.

While all of this was happening, I was struggling with an auto-immune condition that no one could identify. I had eczema all over my body. After I had Simon, the eczema got worse. One night, I cried myself to sleep. My body was on fire. My husband was draping wet towels all over me. It was the only thing that offered even a bit of soothing relief. We started considering moving to Florida because tanning seemed to help with the Vitamin D. I had all these things I was trying to piece together, and I just couldn't. When I was 23, I was diagnosed with Rheumatoid Arthritis. I was in my junior year of nursing school and I could not write notes because it hurt my joints so badly. I got myself an iPad and laptop to do everything I could digitally. Holding a pencil was way too much.

I was overweight. I had this terrible bleeding eczema all over my body. I had tried everything. I had used steroids. I tried Chinese medicine. I tried silver. If I thought it would help eczema, I bought it. I spent thousands of dollars. Some remedies might help for a short time, but if I ever went a day without it, the symptoms would creep right back. I was exercising and eating healthy, but not losing the weight. I found a detox program online. I decided since I'd heard a lot of people lose a lot of weight on detox, I bought it.

The program was a 21-day detox, where you take some supplements and they tell you what to eat every single day. At the end of the detox, the end of the 3 weeks, I was finally seeing some relief for the first time in my life from the eczema. It was almost gone. It was interesting because I wasn't doing anything topically. I didn't realize it, I was just working on my gut and my insides. Two weeks later I had a period for the first time in months. Two weeks after that I conceived my daughter. During pregnancy your immune system is suppressed so things tend to go better for those with auto-immune challenges. After I had my daughter, I was thinking "ok, there is something to this detox thing."

As a nurse working in labor and delivery, I was used to the medical mindset and pharmacology practices. I was stuck with the mindset of taking a drug for a condition. I didn't like the drugs they gave me; often they made me feel worse. I couldn't find anything else that would work. I thought I was stuck.

I remembered the eczema had gone away with the detox. I was starting to connect the dots. However, I felt like I couldn't be living in a state of detox all the time. I went to a conference. The man who had created the detox was there. I asked him about the idea of living in a state of detox. He told me it was possible. There are ways to support your body through supplementation to keep the inflammation at bay. Inflammation. There was another dot. I did another detox and felt fantastic. This was the only time I'd lose weight quickly and the eczema would go away. I was doing research and found there was a connection between eczema and gut health. There's something to this gut health thing. I was determined to get healthy.

I've always been transparent about my journey on Facebook. One day, someone reached out to me and told me about this gut protocol and invited me to do it with them. It was a thousand-dollar program plus the supplements. I was desperate. While I was doing this gut healing program, someone else reached out to me and asked if I'd ever heard of Dr. Patrick and The Wellness Way. I was in the middle of the program. I had spent over $1000 on this gut thing; I was going to stick with it. They were relentless "he really makes the connections when he talks about your gut health, he talks about how it affects your hormones, inflammation, everything." All I could think was it's all connected! It's not just gut = eczema, it's gut = hormones and eczema and I have all these things going on. Maybe it all originates in my gut!

I was seeing some results from the gut protocol, but not like I wanted for how much I had paid. I called to set up an appointment with Dr. Patrick. I remember sitting in the waiting room thinking "Either these people are going to be a bunch of weirdos and totally out there or there's going to be something to this. I'm about to find out. They took my x-rays and showed me the inflammation in my gut. They actually *showed* me the inflammation in my gut! Dots connected. I talked with Dr. Patrick and told him my story. I had brought in my giant tub of supplements that I was taking. His response, "there's nothing wrong with these supplements but how do you know they are the ones you need?" All I could say was, "I don't know, it's just part of the protocol." He showed me the problem with the protocol. It wasn't individualized to each person. That's why I wasn't getting the results I was looking for. He started to help me shift my mind and think differently. I went to the Inflammation Talk the next day. Finally, it clicked. The Wellness Way Clinics offer Inflammation Talks every couple of weeks for new patients. This talk is the foundation and introduces new patients to their approach. Inflammation is the key to all sources of disease and dysfunction within the body. This is what I had been looking for. I had been researching for years trying to find answers and connect the dots between my gut, eczema, auto-immune conditions and PCOS. I finally found someone who could put those connections together!

After the Inflammation Talk, I boldly approached Dr. Patrick. The only thing I could think was, "if there's anything I am going to do, I have to work for this guy. I have to learn everything he knows." I said, "I don't know if you remember me. I was in as a new patient yesterday. I had mentioned that I am a nurse. Your Inflammation Talk opened my eyes. I finally get it. Women's hormones and autoimmune conditions are my passion; it's something I have struggled with. I really think this approach could apply to infertility for women across the country and I want to be an expert. Would you consider bringing me on board?" His response was quick, "Yes, come in for an interview." I was totally blown away. "REALLY?" I'm not typically that bold, but there was something inside me. I knew I couldn't leave without addressing it.

I went in for the interview. The timing was perfect. The clinic in Green Bay, WI was looking for a nurse to help with the IV center. It was a great way to get trained and see what happens at The Wellness Way. My wellness journey began. I recognized the difference between The Wellness Way Approach and the traditional medical model. The allopathic medical model sees a list of symptoms and comes up with a diagnosis to treat. They don't look at the whole picture. It didn't resonate with me that I'd have to live a life constantly relying on medication or supplements like others suggested. I felt like I should be able to fix it. Medication or supplements should be part time. The

Wellness Way looks at things differently and looks at people as individuals. I was properly tested; my thyroid, hormone and food allergy test. My food allergy test was eye opening. I discovered I had 42 food allergies. To this day, I have not had anyone come in to the Green Bay clinic with more than me. I started eliminating those immediately. It was very difficult, but necessary. I started taking a few supplements to help with my gut, my iron deficiency and to balance my hormones. Unlike a traditional PCOS patient, I had very low testosterone. A lot of the protocol used in the medical world wouldn't have worked for me; I wouldn't have known why if I hadn't gotten my hormones tested as thoroughly. Within a month of following this new approach, I got my period for the first time in months. It was the first normal period in my life. From then on, I would get it every single month. The first week I lost 10 pounds. I was 80 pounds overweight at that time. Within my first two months I lost over 25 pounds and 80 pounds within the first 6 months. I was feeling like myself again. I had more vitality and energy. Within two months my eczema was completely gone. I was a walking testimony to The Wellness Way Approach!

Everyone had told me I would have auto-immune conditions and take steroids the rest of my life. The Rheumatoid Arthritis, eczema, weight and PCOS were three different systems that were all broken. When I came to The Wellness Way I realized they were connected; they weren't isolated instances. I started sharing my Wellness Way testimony with my friends and have become a great referral source. I soaked up everything I could about hormones and how to balance the body. When my husband and I decided we were ready, we conceived baby #3 the first time we tried. I believe this lifestyle is for everyone. You shouldn't have to take supplements or medication for the rest of your life. Your body can be whole, well, and free of conditions as long as you know and avoid your triggers.

My dreams and desires to reach as many people as I can are becoming a reality. At The Wellness Way, we don't have specialties; everything within the body is connected. However, I have been able to build a practice around this one very special focus. It is so much fun to help women find the root cause of their issues, and then watch them feel so much better like I did. We've had people reach out from all over the world through the power of social media. Women from Switzerland, Argentina, Bhutan, Asia, and England, have found answers.

Every time I share The Wellness Way message, I tell my patients, "you are not broken." A lot of times when women are not able to conceive, it devastates them. It's part of their womanhood; they feel like they are broken. Your body is responding to your environment, we just have to figure out why and fix it. You were created to have babies if that is what you want!

You disagree too! Now what?

Just because the book is done doesn't mean this story is over. We are growing with multiple voices saying, "I disagree." We are a movement. Share your #Idisagree story with us and make your voice heard! Connect with us on our social channels and website. Follow-up with a clinic near you to attend their events and sign up to get some insights as a patient. We have a lot to offer, and are excited to keep empowering you to think differently, and say I Disagree!

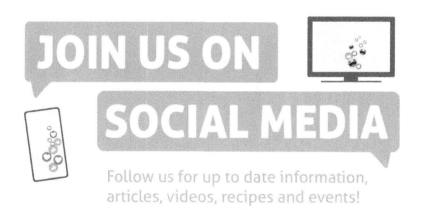

JOIN US ON SOCIAL MEDIA

Follow us for up to date information, articles, videos, recipes and events!

     The Wellness Way
Dr. Patrick Flynn

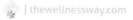 thewellnessway.com

Made in the USA
Monee, IL
14 October 2023

44590984R10116